Human Insulin by Tryptic Transpeptidations of Porcine Insulin and Biosynthetic Precursors

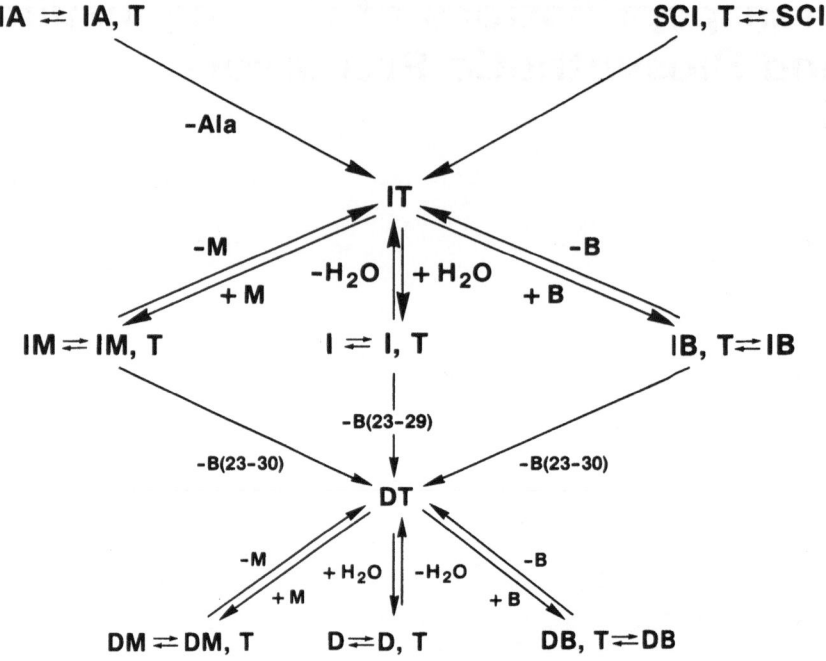

Human Insulin by Tryptic Transpeptidations of Porcine Insulin and Biosynthetic Precursors

Jan Markussen

WKAP ARCHIEF

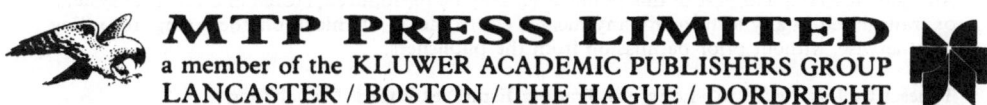

MTP PRESS LIMITED
a member of the KLUWER ACADEMIC PUBLISHERS GROUP
LANCASTER / BOSTON / THE HAGUE / DORDRECHT

Denne afhandling er af Danmarks Tekniske Højskole antaget til forsvar for den tekniske doktorgrad.

Antagelsen er sket efter bedømmelse af den foreliggende afhandling og 9 artikler, ref. 1, 65, 69, 70, 71, 86, 87, 89 og 112 i referencelisten, pagina 103–108.

Lyngby, den 24. juni 1987.

Hans Peter Jensen
Rektor

/Paul Carpentier
Administrationschef

This thesis has been accepted by the Technical University of Denmark for public defense in fulfilment of the requirements for the Degree of Doctor Technices.

The acceptance is based on this dissertation and 9 papers, ref. 1, 65, 69, 70, 71, 86, 87, 89, 112, in the list of literature, page 103–108.

Lyngby, June 24, 1987.

Hans Peter Jensen
President

/Paul Carpentier
Secretary

Published in the UK and Europe by
MTP Press Limited
Falcon House
Lancaster, England

British Library Cataloguing in Publication Data

Markussen, Jan
  Human insulin by tryptic transpeptidations of porcine insulin and biosynthetic precursors.
  1. Insulin
  I. Title
  615'.365   RS431.I/

  ISBN-13: 978-0-7462-0059-9   e-ISBN-13: 978-94-009-3187-9
  DOI: 10.1007/978-94-009-3187-9

Published in the USA by
MTP Press
A division of Kluwer Academic Publishers
101 Philip Drive
Norwell, MA 02061, USA

Typeset by Lasertext Ltd., Longford Trading Estate, Stretford, Manchester.
Printed by Butler and Tanner Ltd., Frome and London.

Contents

Acknowledgements

The present work on transpeptidation of porcine insulin and biosynthetic precursors was carried out in the research laboratories of Novo Industri A/S. Many of my colleagues within Novo have made contributions, for which I am grateful.

Threonine esters were synthesized by B. Lundt, F. Grønvald and H. Petersen. Immobilized trypsin preparations were made by S. Gestrilius. Genes coding for the biosynthetic precursors were synthesized, inserted in plasmids and expressed in yeast by F. Norris, K. Norris and M. T. Hansen.

Fermentations on pilot-scale were conducted by I. Diers and the preparative work-up by H. O. Voigt.

On the analytical side, water content was analysed by R. Amsler, amino acid composition by M. Christensen, amino acid sequences by L. Thim. HPLC separation of human insulin and des-(B30) insulin was carried out by L. Snel.

J. Villumsen was helpful in the mathematical analysis of specificity, Chapter 3, by solving the differential equations. Å. Vølund participated in establishing the kinetic models; he wrote the first program we used for simulation of reaction progress and conducted simulations with this program as well as with the acquired program KINSIM. He also participated in the stimulating discussions with B. Lautrup and M. Ålund of Scientific Consulting in the painstaking attempts to make the analog computer, MOSES, simulate the reaction progress. The program that eventually was found to simulate reaction progress fastest and most satisfactorily was developed by B. Lautrup and M. Ålund. Its execution requires only a personal computer. K. Schaumburg of the H.C. Ørsted Institute, University of Copenhagen, participated in the planning of the ^{17}O-NMR study and conducted the NMR spectroscopy.

K. H. Jørgensen has, through profound reading of the manuscript, contributed with constructive criticism and suggestions.

The author is grateful to Lone Karakavuk and Bodil Larsen for typing the manuscript and to Kathleen Larsen and Else Jørgensen for linguistic corrections.

A special thanks to my technicians through many years, Lene Drube and Kate Müggler, for precise and reproducible work, loyal collaboration and good spirits.

Copenhagen, June 1986   JAN MARKUSSEN

Abbreviations

A	alanine
A(1–21)	A-chain of insulin
Ac	acetyl
B	Thr(Bu^t)-OBu^t
B(1–29)	B-chain of insulin, residues 1–29
BAEE	N^α-benzoyl-L-arginine ethyl ester
BAPA	N^α-benzoyl-D,L-arginine-p-nitroanilide
BD	1,4-butanediol
Boc	t-butyloxycarbonyl
Boc-OSu	t-butyloxycarbonyl-N-hydroxy succinimide
Bu^t	t-butyl ether
Bz	benzoyl
D	desoctapeptide-(B23–B30) insulin
DAI	des(AlaB30) porcine insulin
DCC	dicyclohexylcarbodiimide
Dhch	1,2-dihydroxycyclohex-1,2-ylene
Disc electrophoresis	discontinuous (pH) electrophoresis
DMAC	N,N-dimethylacetamide
DMF	N,N-dimethylformamide
DMSO	dimethyl sulphoxide
DOI	desoctapeptide-(B23-B30) insulin
DOI-B	Thr^{B23}(Bu^t)-OBu^t, desheptapeptide-(B24–B30) insulin
DOI-M	Thr^{B23}-OMe, desheptapeptide-(B24–B30) insulin
DOI-SB	Thr^{B23}-OBu^t, desheptapeptide-(B24–B30) insulin
EDTA	ethylenediaminetetraacetic acid
FC	first crystal crop
G	Gibb's free energy
GuCl	guanidinium hydrochloride
HI	human insulin
HI(Bu^t)-OBu^t	Thr^{B30}(Bu^t)-OBu^t human insulin
HI-OBu^t	Thr^{B30}-OBu^t human insulin
HI-OMe	Thr^{B30}-OMe human insulin
HI-OR	Thr^{B30}-OR human insulin
HMPA	hexamethylphosphoramide
HOAc	acetic acid

HOBt	1-hydroxybenzotriazole
HOSu	N-hydroxy succinimide
HPLC	high pressure liquid chromatography
I	des-(B30) insulin
IA	porcine insulin
IB	$Thr^{B30}(Bu^t)$-OBu^t human insulin
IM	Thr^{B30}-OMe human insulin
ISB	Thr^{B30}-OBu^t human insulin
IT	des-(B30) insulinyl^{B29}-trypsin
I,T	des-(B30) insulin, trypsin association complex
IThr	human insulin
k	first order rate constant
k_2	rate constant for enzyme acylation
k_3	rate constant for acyl-enzyme deacylation
k_a	second-order rate constant for autolysis
K	lysine
K_e	equilibrium constant
$K_e(DB)$	equilibrium constant for $D + B \rightleftharpoons DB$
$K_e(DM)$	equilibrium constant for $D + M \rightleftharpoons DM$
$K_e(IB)$	equilibrium constant for $I + B \rightleftharpoons IB$
$K_e(IM)$	equilibrium constant for $I + M \rightleftharpoons IM$
$K_e(ISB)$	equilibrium constant for $I + SB \rightleftharpoons ISB$
$K_e(ITmb)$	equilibrium constant for $I + Thr$-$OTmb \rightleftharpoons I$-$Thr$-$Tmb$
K.F.	Karl Fischer method for water analysis
K_I; K_{IA}, K_{IM}, K_{IB}	equilibrium constants for trypsin association, e.g. $IM:IM + T \rightleftharpoons IM, T$
K_m	Michaelis–Menten constant
M	molar; Thr-OMe
Mse	methylsulphonylethyl
$N(Et)_3$	triethyl amine
NMM	N-methyl morpholine
NMP	N-methyl-2-pyrrolidone
OAc^-	acetate
OBu	butan-1-ol ester
OBu^t	t-butyl ester
OMe	methyl ester
PAGE	polyacrylamide gel electrophoresis
PEG	polyethylene glycol
PI	porcine insulin
PTH	phenylthiohydantoin
q	specificity = ratio between two rate constants
R	arginine; gas constant
RP-HPLC	reverse phase HPLC
S	serine
SB	Thr-OBu^t
SCI	single-chain des-(B30) insulin
SCI(ss)	single-chain des-(B30) insulin, semisynthetic
SCI(ge)	single-chain des-(B30) insulin, genetic engineering

SCI-AAK	B(1–29)-A-A-K-A(1–21) insulin
SCI-SK	B(1–29)-S-K-A(1–21) insulin
T	trypsin; concentration of trypsin; absolute temperature
TC	twice crystallized
TFA	trifluoroacetic acid
THF	tetrahydrofuran
Tmb	trimethylbenzyl
TPCK	L-(1-tosylamide-2-phenyl)ethyl chloromethyl ketone
Tris	tris(hydroxymethyl)methylamine
Z	benzyloxycarbonyl

1
Introduction and background

1. SCENARIO AND SCOPE

The present studies were initiated by events that took place in August–September, 1979. Morihara and co-workers published in August a paper in *Nature* describing a simple two-step method to convert porcine insulin into human insulin via des(Ala^{B30}) porcine insulin. At the Second International Insulin Symposium in Aachen in September, H. G. Gattner and co-workers presented a very similar method. Furthermore, R. Chance from the Eli Lilly company confirmed that the preliminary reports from Genentech on fermentation of insulin A- and B-chains in *E. coli* were factual and that chain combinations rendering insulin in fair yields had been carried through successfully.

In the first phase of the present studies emphasis was put on the conversion of porcine insulin to human insulin in a technical and economically justifiable process. For competitive reasons a veritable race to be the first to launch human insulin developed between the E. Lilly and Novo companies, culminating with the launch of Novo's 'semisynthetic' human insulin in England, June 9th, 1982 and E. Lilly's 'biosynthetic' human insulin in England, September 16th, 1982[1]. The 'biosynthetic' insulin had an element of semisynthesis involved, namely the A- and B-chain combination substantially improved for the purpose by R. Chance *et al.*[2].

The semisynthetic human insulin was produced by a one-step conversion of porcine insulin in an organic–aqueous medium in a process invented by the author. The process termed transpeptidation is technically more attractive than the two-step process by Morihara *et al.* The first such transpeptidation was carried out November 12th, 1979. Compositions of reaction mixtures were at first analysed by disc electrophoresis, from January, 1980 by RP-HPLC. By February 29th, 1980 yields of 95–97% had been reached, a satisfactory result considering that some impurities like porcine proinsulin were converted into human insulin ester along with porcine insulin; impurities that due to their immunogenicity are removed from purified porcine insulin. Human insulin of porcine insulin origin became the first naturally occurring protein to be manufactured by semisynthesis. Since the starting material,

1

porcine insulin, is limited, it was of vital interest to carry out the conversion reaction with close to quantitative yields. During this work it became the intention of the author to understand the influence of the various factors on the yield causatively; was a low yield due to an unfavourable thermodynamic equilibrium, to untimely enzyme inactivation/denaturation, or to irreversible by-product formation?

Transpeptidation is defined as a replacement reaction, in which one of the components of a peptide bond is replaced by another, rendering a new peptide bond. The transpeptidation reaction needs catalysis by an enzyme. Trypsin was and is the enzyme of choice because it is inexpensive, available in a highly purified form and specific for lysine and arginine. Porcine pancreatic trypsin is particularly attractive, as its use does not add any new contaminants to human insulin that are not removed by existing purification methods used in the manufacture of monocomponent porcine insulin.

The use of trypsin in the transpeptidation reaction gives rise to by-products when reaction takes place at Arg^{B22}, namely desoctapeptide-B(23–30) insulin and its threonine esters in position B23, DOI-Thr-OR, both biologically inactive. The control of transpeptidation reactions using trypsin is the topic of Chapter 4. Specific transpeptidation would have been much easier if the lysine-specific *Achromobacter lyticus* protease had been available at a modest price. A few examples have been included to show the superiority of this enzyme over trypsin in the transpeptidation of single-chain des-(B30) insulin to human insulin ester.

Tryptic transpeptidations of insulins in organic–aqueous media are slow reactions, not especially suited for mechanistic enzymology studies. Consequently, adaptation to the generally accepted acyl-enzyme theory for serine proteases is made, and the kinetic studies in Chapter 6 are interpreted using common Michaelis-Menten kinetics, despite dissociations being so large that K_m values cannot be determined. A pronounced inhibition of transpeptidation was found whenever Thr-OMe was present, and a kinetic model accounting for this inhibition is provided in Chapter 6.

In the second phase of the present studies the transpeptidation method was brought into use in the conversion of biosynthetic single-chain insulin precursors into human insulin esters, a step in an alternative process for biosynthetic insulin rendering the A- and B-chain combination *in vitro* superfluous. The disulphide bridges of insulin have been formed in yeast during fermentation and are present in the single-chain precursors. Transpeptidation of biosynthetic single-chain insulin precursors to an ester of human insulin will eventually replace the transpeptidation of porcine insulin in the manufacture of human insulin. It proved more difficult to open up the tightly knotted single-chain precursors selectively with trypsin at Lys^{B29} without side-reaction at Arg^{B22} than to transpeptidize porcine insulin at Lys^{B29}, meaning that steric hindrance had been introduced at Lys^{B29} by connecting Lys^{29} to Gly^{A1}, both when bound directly and through a few amino acid residues. The search for conditions specific enough to permit such transpeptidations was completed December, 1984, when yields of 90% had been reached. These reactions are the topic of Chapter 5. As specificity of the transpeptidations is a problem in general, a definition of specificity and a simple model is introduced in Chapter 3 in order to handle the data of Chapter 4 and 5.

Focus is placed on the transpeptidation reactions. Methods for recovering the products after reaction will be referred to, but are outside the scope of this treatise. Insulin derivatives substituted in position B30 are mentioned (section 7) only because the syntheses enlighten the mechanism of transpeptidations at Lys^{B29}, whereas neither the properties of B30 substituted insulins nor of human insulin will be dealt with.

The clinical benefit from using human insulin instead of porcine insulin was expected to be a decreased immunological response. The immunogenicity of the highly purified monocomponent porcine insulin is already very low, so it was anticipated that a reduction of immunogenicity would be very difficult to prove. Consequently, newly diagnosed, insulin-dependent, diabetic children were chosen for the clinical trials, as children are known to respond more vigorously than adults to an immunological challenge. A total of 135 patients were randomly allocated at diagnosis of diabetes to treatment with either porcine or human insulin in a double-blind trial conducted in Scandinavia. Levels of antibodies (IgG) binding to insulin were significantly lower in the group treated with human insulin after 3 and 12 months of therapy[3].

Allergic reactions to insulin have become rare as the purity of insulins has improved. It was found that some patients with established insulin allergy could be treated with human insulin without allergic reactions[4].

In order to improve insulin therapy Novo is currently substituting porcine insulin with human insulin in a large number of countries. Clinical trials of human insulin, prepared from a single-chain precursor produced in yeast, were started at the beginning of June, 1986.

2. PEPTIDE BOND SYNTHESIS USING PROTEASES

The hydrolysis of a peptide bond by a protease may be written as a sequence of two reactions, first the enzyme catalysed uptake of water (i) and secondly a proton transfer from the formed carboxylic acid to the amino group, neutralization (ii):

(i) $\qquad R_1\text{-CO-NH-}R_2 + H_2O \rightleftharpoons R_1COOH + NH_2R_2$

(ii) $\qquad R_1COOH + NH_2R_2 \rightleftharpoons R\text{-COO}^- + NH_3^+\text{-}R_2$

The first law of thermodynamics predicts that an enzyme catalysing a reaction in one direction must also catalyse the reverse reaction; otherwise we could construct a type 1 perpetuum mobile with the enzyme acting as the Maxwell demon. The reversal of hydrolysis is consequently not a question of enzyme specificity. Since peptide bond hydrolysis runs spontaneously under physiological conditions, meaning that the change in free Gibb's energy, ΔG, is negative, the reversal of hydrolysis requires either a change of conditions or a coupling to energy-delivering processes in order to make ΔG negative. Energy-yielding processes may be physicochemical in nature,

3

e.g. removal of the peptide product from solution and concentration of the solution. Examples of energy-coupling by chemical means are activation of the carboxylic acid as an ester or amide and removal of the product from the equilibrium by another enzyme, rendering a new product inaccessible to the enzyme that establishes the equilibrium. The energy-coupling process may influence the chemical potential of either substrates or product, 'the horse either pushes or pulls the waggon'.

When energy is provided by activation of the carboxyl acid component, e.g. by ester formation, the product peptide is still substrate for the protease and hydrolysis occurs. If hydrolysis is slow compared to peptide synthesis from the activated carboxylic acid, preparative peptide synthesis with a time-dependent yield has been achieved, viz. kinetically controlled synthesis. When free energy is provided by changes of the conditions in the medium that shift the equilibria (i) and (ii), the result is a thermodynamically controlled peptide synthesis, with a time-independent yield after attainment of equilibrium. Examples of both are plentiful from the late 1930s to the early 1950s, a period when much work was put into elucidating the possible role of proteases for the synthesis of proteins. The transpeptidation reactions of porcine insulin and biosynthetic precursors using trypsin result in equilibria like (i) and (ii), making them thermodynamically controlled reactions. It will be appropriate to treat the thermodynamics before citing selected examples of peptide bond synthesis using proteases.

The overall formation of a peptide bond (iii) has an apparent equilibrium constant K_{syn}, where ΣA and ΣB indicate total concentrations of ionized and non-ionized forms of A and B.

(iii) $$\Sigma A + \Sigma B \rightleftharpoons A\text{-}B + H_2O; \quad K_{syn} = \frac{[A\text{-}B][H_2O]}{[\Sigma A][\Sigma B]}$$

In diluted aqueous solutions the activity of water may be defined equal to unity. However, when the water concentration is reduced, e.g. by addition of organic solvents, the expression (iii), including the water concentration term, serves the purpose of describing the changes best.

The carboxylic acid A and the ammonium form of the amine B dissociate according to (iv) and (v):

(iv) $$A \rightleftharpoons A^- + H^+; \quad K_A = \frac{[A^-][H^+]}{[A]}$$

(v) $$BH^+ \rightleftharpoons B + H^+; \quad K_B = \frac{[B][H^+]}{[BH^+]}$$

The non-ionized forms A and B condense under peptide bond formation, the equilibrium constant K_c being defined by (vi):

(vi) $$A + B \rightleftharpoons A\text{-}B + H_2O; \quad K_c = \frac{[A\text{-}B][H_2O]}{[A][B]}$$

ΣA and ΣB may be eliminated from (iii) using (iv), (v) and (vi), inserting

$\Sigma A = A + A^-$ and $\Sigma B = B + BH^+$. The elimination converts (iii) into (vii):

(vii) $\qquad\qquad K_{syn} = K_c/(1 + K_A/H^+ + H^+/K_B + K_A/K_B)$

When pK_A and pK_B are far apart and $pK_A \ll pH \ll pK_B$ ($K_A \gg H^+ \gg K_B$) the three first terms of the denominator vanish compared to K_A/K_B and (vii) transforms into the simpler form (viii):

(viii) $\qquad\qquad K_{syn} = K_c \times K_B/K_A$

K_{syn} is practically independent of pH in a broad range between pK_A and pK_B, approximately 1 pH unit from the pK values. A change of conditions that makes K_A and K_B approach each other effects an increase in K_{syn}.

In the general case the influence of pH on K_{syn} is given by (vii). K_{syn} is at a maximum when $H^+ = \sqrt{K_A \times K_B}$ or $pH = (pK_A + pK_B)/2$. If pK_B becomes smaller than pK_A, K_{syn} is still at maximum at $pH = (pK_A + pK_B)/2$, the upper limit of K_{syn} being equality to K_c as the inequality $pK_B < pK_A$ increases. In the special case where $pH = pK_A = pK_B$, K_{syn} equals $K_c/4$.

When the reacting groups of A and B have ionizable groups in the vicinity, the state of charge of these affects pK_A and pK_B, as in zwitterions of free amino acids. The function of K_{syn} shows two maxima at pH about pK_A and pK_B, cf. Borsook[5] and Carpenter[6].

Using heat capacity[7] and heat of combustion measurements[8], Huffman calculated the changes in standard free energy in the hydrolysis of peptide bonds, defining the standard state of reactants as the solid state except for water. Values ranging from $-6\,kJ/mole$ (Bz-Gly) to $-16\,kJ/mole$ (Ala-Gly) were found.

The change in free energy from the standard state in solution where the activities of reactants are put at unity, ΔG_0, is given by (ix):

(ix) $\qquad\qquad \Delta G_0 = -RT\ln K_{syn}; \quad \Delta G_0 = \Delta G_0 c + \Delta G_0 n$

The concept to separate ΔG_0 in a term for the condensation between non-ionized reactants, $\Delta G_0 c$, and a term for the reversal of the neutralisation, $\Delta G_0 n$, was introduced by Linderstrøm-Lang[9]. Using Huffman's calorimetric data for ΔG_s (substances in solid state except water), solubility data, acid-base dissociation constants and activity coefficients, he divided ΔG_0 for the overall reaction into the neutralization and condensation terms. Whereas $\Delta G_0 n$ was positive and varied considerably dependent upon the pK values of reactants and products, nearly constant and negative values were found for $\Delta G_0 c$, ranging from -19 to $-25\,kJ/mole$. That $\Delta G_0 c$ is negative means that reaction (vi) at reasonable concentrations of A and B will be displaced towards peptide bond synthesis. The large positive contributions from $\Delta G_0 n$ render ΔG_0 positive and cause the overall reaction to be displaced towards hydrolysis. Values of $\Delta G_0 n$ vary from $38\,kJ/mole$ in the most unfavourable case, viz. formation of Gly-Gly from glycine, to $30\,kJ/mole$ for formation of hippuric acid from benzoic acid and glycine and to $23\,kJ/mole$ for the formation of Bz-Gly-Gly from benzoic acid and diglycine. For peptide bond formation in the favourable case, where none of the reactants are zwitterions, ΔG_0 was estimated to be $4.9\,kJ/mole$ (Ac-Gly + Gly-OMe). Dobry et al.[10] measured ΔG_0 for the synthesis of Bz-Tyr-Gly-NH_2 from Bz-Tyr and

5

Gly-NH$_2$ to be 1.8 kJ/mole, using isotope dilution analysis to study the equilibrium. Carpenter[6] elaborated on the separation of the terms of ΔG_0 and introduced a non-ionized compound convention: 'the standard free energy change on hydrolysis at a specified temperature refers to the free energy change involved in the hydrolysis of non-ionized reactant at unit activity in water by water in the liquid state to yield non-ionized products at unit activity in water'. Using thermochemical data he estimated $\Delta G_0 c$ to be -20 ± 3 kJ/mole, in good agreement with Linderstrøm-Lang's estimates. Due to 'the limitations in accuracy of the combustion and entropy data, as well as some of the assumptions made in the use of activity coefficients and ionization constants, the observed spread of values of $\Delta G_0 c$ of peptide bonds is probably well within the range of experimental error'.

Combination of (vii) and (ix) leads to (x):

(x) $\quad \Delta G_0 = -RT \ln K_c + RT \ln(1 + K_A/H^+ + H^+/K_B + K_A/K_B)$

The first term signifies the changes in ΔG_0 that are influenced by the activities of the reacting molecules, the second term the concentration variations due to ionization of reactants. In the simple case where $K_A \gg H^+ \gg K_B$ we derive (xi):

(xi) $\qquad \Delta G_0 = -2.3 RT(\log K_c + pK_A - pK_B)$

The most powerful means to decrease $\Delta pK = pK_B - pK_A$, and hence to increase $-\Delta G_0$, is to add organic solvents to the medium. Michaelis and Mizutani[11] in 1925 described the decrease in the dissociation constants of acids with increasing concentrations of ethanol. The pH in a mixture was defined as that of an aqueous solution giving rise to the same potential as measured with a hydrogen electrode, i.e. liquid-junction potentials were ignored. They found that the changes in dissociation constants were quite similar for various carboxylic acids, about 2 pH units upwards for the shift from water to 80% ethanol. The dissociation constants of the ammonium form of amines were less sensitive to changes from water to ethanol/water mixtures, the change in pK typically being about 0.5 pH unit downwards for the shift from water to 80% ethanol[11,12].

The effect was utilized by Butler and Reithel[13] in the synthesis of urea from ammonium carbonate by urease in water mixed with glycerol or 1,2-propandiol, and by Homandberg et al.[14] in the resynthesis of the Arg-Ile bond of split soybean trypsin inhibitor by trypsin and in the synthesis of Z-Trp-Gly-NH$_2$ from Z-Trp and Gly-NH$_2$ by chymotrypsin. The shift in equilibrium towards synthesis by changing from water to 60% glycerol or 80% 1,4-butanediol was much larger than the change in water concentration, as accounted for in the term K_c above, could explain. It was concluded that the major cause in the shift of the equilibria toward peptide bond synthesis upon addition of organic solvents is the increase in the pK of the reactant carboxyl group, resulting in a shift of equilibrium (iv) toward the left. With this, at least semiquantitatively correct argument, the concepts for the use of proteases in peptide formation in organic media were available, and immediately put to use in insulin chemistry, vide section 3.

6

Homandberg et al.[14] measured pK_A (Ac-Gly) and pK_B (Gly-NH$_2$) potentiometrically in 80% of a variety of organic solvents. Whereas pK_B varied less than 0.2 pH unit between solvents, large and varying increases in pK_A were observed. The errors due to improper pH calibration in the solvent/water mixtures are cancelled in the determinations of ΔpK values. The shift in $-\Delta Gn$ by changing from water to a mixture of organic solvent and water, $\Delta(-\Delta Gn)$, may be approximated using (xi), assuming $pK_B \gg pH \gg pK_A$ and that activity coefficients of reactants remain constant (xii):

(xii) $\Delta(-\Delta Gn) = 2.3\,RT(\Delta pK(H_2O) - \Delta pK(mixture)) = 2.3\,RT\Delta\Delta pK$

As a result of the approach of pK_A to pK_B by the addition of organic solvents, the broad pH-optimum for K_{syn} narrows, and the importance of selecting pH $= (pK_A + pK_B)/2$ increases. In 60% triethylene glycol the pH range for optimal K_{syn} for the coupling of Z-Trp to Gly-NH$_2$ covers about 1 pH unit. The increase in pK_A by addition of organic co-solvents can only partly be explained by increased electrostatic interactions between the oppositely charged ions displacing equation (iv) to the left, because the $\Delta\Delta pK$ values do not correlate to the dielectric constants of the solvents. The ranking of solvents according to $\Delta\Delta pK$ values in 80% of various solvents in water was:

DMSO (3.49) > dioxan (2.13) > acetone (2.09) > acetonitrile = BD

   = 1,5-pentanediol (1.55) > ethanol (1.53) > ethylene glycol (1.23)

   > glycerol (0.88).

When the amino component is a weak base like aniline (pK = 4.6), the equilibrium is favourably displaced towards peptide bond synthesis. However, the described anilide syntheses involve a displacement of (vi) due to precipitation of the product from the aqueous solution. The success of the precipitation method depends upon whether the solubility limit of the product can be reached with a given $-\Delta G_0$ while keeping the carboxylic acid and amino component in solution. This is often the case when forming dipeptides from amino acids protected by hydrophobic groups.

Other causes than electrostatic forces, 'solvation effects', e.g. hydrogen bonding and entropy effects, may contribute to the decrease of carboxylic acid dissociation in organic co-solvents. The increase in $-\Delta Gn$ of about 19 kJ/mole in 80% DMSO suffices to bring about high-yield synthesis between single charged reactants, provided the reactants A and B are present in concentrations of about 1 M. If yields are calculated on the basis of one of the reactants (the expensive one), high-yield syntheses are achieved provided the other is present in substantial concentration. The increase in $-\Delta Gc$ due to the decrease in water by a factor 5 amounts to 4 kJ/mole, provided the activity coefficients remain constant, demonstrating the much smaller contribution from the $-\Delta Gc$ term than from the $-\Delta Gn$ term. In 80% glycerol the two terms become approximately equal.

Ideally, the effect of solvents on $\Delta(-\Delta Gc)$ should include the changes in activity coefficients of A, B, A-B and water. The activity coefficient of water

7

depends on interactions with the particular solvent. Such interactions tend to decrease the chemical potential of water and thus further promote peptide bond synthesis.

The effect of adding strong electrolytes to a solution of ions is a decrease of the chemical potentials of the ions. In diluted aqueous solutions the activity coefficients for monovalent ions decrease with the ionic strength I according to (xiii):

$$(xiii) \qquad -\log f = \text{const.} \sqrt{I} \sim 0.5 \sqrt{I}$$

Decreasing the chemical potentials of the ions A^- and BH^+ causes an unfavourable displacement of equation (ii) toward ionization. Other salts than those derived from buffering A/B with a suitable base/acid should be avoided. Homandberg et al.[14] observed a decrease in K_{syn} by a factor 2 by raising the concentration of NaCl from 0 to 0.75 M in 60% triethylene glycol, a smaller change than predicted from the approximation (xiii), valid only for dilute solutions of salts.

Removal of the product by complexation is another way to promote synthesis in an energetically impossible situation. Sealock and Laskowski[15] coupled arginine to des(Arg^{64}) split soybean trypsin inhibitor ($K_{syn} = 10^{-2}$ M^{-1}) by carboxypeptidase B in the presence of trypsin (stability constant $= 10^8\,M^{-1}$), rendering synthesis of split and genuine soybean trypsin inhibitor–trypsin complex with an overall K_{syn} of $10^6\,M^{-2}$. Energy is, of course, required to dissociate the complex subsequent to synthesis, e.g. by a drop in pH.

Kowalski et al.[16] used complexation with chymotrypsin instead of trypsin and coupling by carboxypeptidase A instead of carboxypeptidase B to couple tryptophan to des(Arg^{63}) split soybean trypsin inhibitor (previous notation 64) and thus converted the soybean trypsin inhibitor to a chymotrypsin inhibitor. Likewise, phenylalanine could be substituted in position 63 whereas an attempt to introduce leucine failed, possibly due to an inadequate stability constant of Leu^{63} soybean inhibitor–chymotrypsin complex. Furthermore, they coupled split, inactivated soybean trypsin inhibitor at Arg^{63} to Gly-NH_2 in 3 M Gly-NH_2 by trypsin in a yield of about 50% corresponding to $\Delta G_0 = 2.7\,kJ/mole$, in fair agreement with the value[10] for coupling of Bz-Tyr to Gly-NH_2.

In the kinetically controlled synthesis free energy is provided to make $-\Delta G$ positive. The most commonly used method of activation is to introduce the carboxylic acid component as an ester, amide or peptide. An intermediate, the acyl-enzyme, is formed, the linkage from the carbonyl group going to the oxygen of the serine (serine proteases) or to the sulphur of the cysteine (thiol proteases) of the active sites of the respective enzymes, e.g. for serine proteases (xiv):

$$(xiv) \qquad R_1\text{-COOR} + \text{HO-enzyme} \rightarrow R_1\text{-CO-O-enzyme} + \text{ROH}$$

A competitive partition between water and the amino component results in either hydrolysis or peptide bond formation (xv):

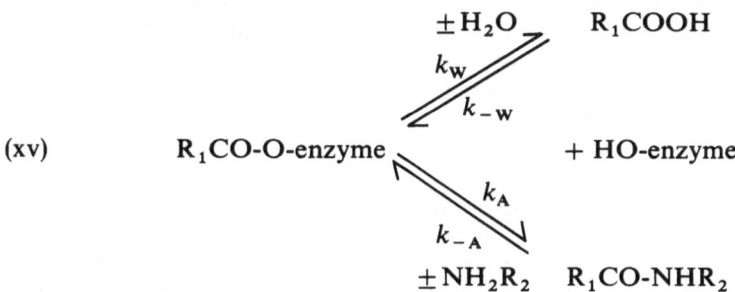

(xv)

If neither water nor amino component binds to the enzyme prior to deacylation, the initial ratio between the desired peptide ($R_1CO-NHR_2$) and by-product (R_1-COOH) is given by $k_A[NH_2R_2]/k_W[H_2O]$.

As primary amino groups usually are much better nucleophiles than water, the initial ratio is often high even if the water concentration is high compared to that of the amino component. The product gives rise to acyl-enzyme formation at a rate proportional to $k_{-A}[R_1CO-NH-R_2]$, so the ratio between product and by-product decreases with time. At the appropriate time, when the yield is at maximum, the reaction is stopped.

Bender et al.[17] observed a simple partition between water and methanol in the deacylation of trans-cinnamoyl-α-chymotrypsin, in that the rate of methanolysis increased proportionally to the concentration of methanol, without saturation of the enzyme by methanol at some stage. This implies that neither water nor methanol binds to the acyl-enzyme before deacylation. Later Fink and Bender[18], by studying the papain-catalysed hydrolysis of p-nitrophenyl N-acetyl-L-tryptophanate in the presence of 1-pentanol, arrived at the conclusion that the added nucleophile binds to papain in two different sites. One site may be identical to S_1', i.e. the one binding the substrate leaving group P_1'. The other influences K_m and k_2, i.e. the acylation reaction. With 1-pentanol occupying the S_1', binding site hydrolysis appears to be blocked, pointing at a necessity for binding and orientation of water prior to hydrolysis in or near the S_1' site. Further evidence for binding of the nucleophile in the S_1' site was provided by Breddam and Ottesen[19]. The aminolysis of Bz-Arg-carboxypeptidase (malt) showed a saturation of the enzyme with Val-NH_2 resulting in a maximum fraction of peptide synthesis of about 0.9, a result incompatible with the simple reaction scheme (xv). Furthermore, a decrease of the acylation reaction rate was observed with increasing concentrations of Val-NH_2 using Bz-Arg-OBu as substrate, indicating competitive inhibition by binding of Val-NH_2 in the S_1' site of malt carboxypeptidase. A similar binding of a nucleophile (Val-NH_2) prior to deacylation of Ac-Tyr-α-chymotrypsin and Bz-Arg-trypsin was demonstrated by Riechmann and Kasche[20], whereas the competitive inhibition of the acylation step by Val-NH_2 was less pronounced.

In the kinetic model proposed in Chapter 6, water and amine component are presumed to compete for binding to the S_1' site, binding being a prerequisite for hydrolysis or aminolysis, respectively. Furthermore, occupancy of water or amine in S_1' is presumed competitively to inhibit binding of substrates possessing the P_1' amino acid residue (transpeptidation), but not substrates missing the P_1' amino acid residue (coupling). The model is simplified as compared to that of Fink and Bender[18], in that a second binding site for nucleophiles, influencing the rate of acylation, has been omitted.

The principle of the kinetically controlled peptide synthesis was used in the studies of Fastrez and Fersht[21] to support the acyl-enzyme mechanism for chymotrypsin. The partition between Ac-Phe and Ac-Phe-Ala-NH$_2$ was studied using Ac-Phe-OMe and Ac-Phe-anilides as substrates. The partition was 1/44 in 1 M Ala-NH$_2$, independent of substrate, strongly suggesting the existence of a common intermediate, the acyl-enzyme. From the mid 1970s the acyl-enzyme intermediate and the charge-relay mechanism have been generally accepted for chymotrypsin, see Blow[22], and it is believed that the same mechanism is conserved in all serine proteases.

There is a clear distinction in the aims of the studies before and after the elucidation of the ribosomal protein synthesis. The older studies aim at clarifying the biological relevance of proteases for the synthesis of proteins, using simpler peptides or amino acids as substrates; in the newer studies emphasis is put on the use of proteases for preparative purposes.

The interest in proteases in connection with protein synthesis dates back to the end of the 19th century. The formation of a precipitate, plastein, when proteases were added to concentrated solutions of peptides, was taken as evidence for peptide bond formation. One preferred model system appears to have been the use of concentrated peptic protein hydrolysates as substrates and pepsin as the enzyme. Additional evidence for protein synthesis was precipitability by trichloroacetic acid, a decrease in free amino nitrogen and an increase in viscosity. The many attempts up to 1930 to prove that plastein indeed represented the result of protein synthesis were reviewed by Wasteneys and Borsook[23]. Linderstrøm-Lang[9] calculated ΔG_0 for the formation of a dipeptide and a long peptide from two shorter peptides to be -1.4 kJ/mole. If the long peptide is sparingly soluble, plastein formation can be explained as a thermodynamically controlled synthesis of peptide bonds. The contradictory finding, viz. the occasional disappearance of the precipitate after some days, can be explained by the presence of other proteases in the enzyme preparation than the one which formed the plastein. This adds an element of kinetics to plastein formation; slow hydrolysis of dissolved plastein and protection of the product against hydrolysis when in the solid phase.

The complex plastein model was eventually left for simpler systems to which rigorous chemical analyses could be applied. Bergmann and Fraenkel-Conrat[24] synthesized Z-Gly-anilide and Bz-Gly-anilide using papain in thermodynamically controlled reactions, favoured by the low pK of aniline and by the insolubility of the anilides in water. Yields of the isolated product were at maximum at pH 4.6, in accordance with the theory predicting optimum at pH $= (pK_A + pK_B)/2$. The rate of synthesis of Bz-Gly-anilide was found to be higher using Bz-Gly-NH$_2$ rather than Bz-Gly-OH as substrate, suggesting a route of synthesis by-passing Bz-Gly-OH, viz. direct replacement of ammonia with aniline. A theory for the replacement of the amino component of a peptide bond was proposed, featuring an intermediate in which the two nitrogen atoms were attached to the carbonyl carbon atom.

Bergmann and Fruton[25] synthesized Bz-Tyr-Gly-anilide from Bz-Tyr and Gly-anilide using chymotrypsin at pH 7.6, whereas the synthesis of the more soluble Bz-Tyr-Gly-NH_2 failed, demonstrating that if $-\Delta G_0$ is too low (pK_B too high) to cause an excess of the solubility of the product, thermo-dynamically controlled peptide bond synthesis might fail. Using papain, Bergmann and Fraenkel-Conrat[26] coupled Bz-Leu to Leu-anilide forming the heavily soluble Bz-Leu-Leu-anilide, whereas the attempt to condense Bz-Leu to Gly-anilide resulted in Bz-Leu-anilide. In the latter case hydrolysis of Gly-anilide must have preceded the synthesis of Bz-Leu-Gly-anilide in concentrations sufficiently high to initiate crystallization.

A simple example of biological significance is the synthesis of hippuric acid. Borsook and Dubnoff[27] calculated ΔG_0 for the condensation of benzoic acid and glycine to 13 kJ/mole by thermodynamic data. Using slices of liver and kidney they were able to convert about 75% of the initially added benzoic acid (0.0025 M) in the presence of 0.01 M glycine, corresponding to a ΔG_0 of about -15 kJ/mole. They realized that this discrepancy could only be explained if the biological hippuric acid synthesis was coupled to an energy-yielding reaction.

One such source of energy, viz. the energy-rich phosphate bonds, was suggested by Lipmann[28] in 1941 as a means to synthesize proteins from amino acids (xvi):

(xvi) $\cdots R\text{-}CO\text{-}OPO_3H_2 + NH_2\text{-}R_1 \cdots \rightarrow \cdots R\text{-}CO\text{-}NH\text{-}R_1 \cdots + H_3PO_4$

The free energy available by decomposition of an energy-rich phosphate bond represents 40–50 kJ/mole, corresponding to a change in K_{syn} of about 2×10^7. Despite Lipmann's precise prediction, the discussions of the likelihood of proteases playing a role in the synthesis of proteins and of the possible energy-yielding mechanisms involved continued to imbue the literature through the 1940s and early 1950s, because the proteases had the unique specificity that was thought necessary in order to explain the syntheses of the highly variable proteins.

Bergmann and Fruton[29] mentioned precipitation as the means by which synthesis possibly is promoted in nature, since some proteins are rather insoluble, e.g. collagen and elastin. They also mentioned linkage to non-protein moieties, e.g. phosphorylation of serine hydroxyl groups. Formation of disulphide bonds and oxidation–reduction reactions were still other possibilities for driving mechanisms. Further speculations on possible energy-coupling mechanisms are found in the reviews by Linderstrøm-Lang[9] and by Borsook and Deasy[30]. Linderstrøm-Lang favours the phosphate ester activation proposed by Lipmann, and both point towards the unlikelihood of transpeptidation by the same enzyme that catalyses hydrolysis, as hydrolysis in many cases appeared to be more rapid than transpeptidation.

Fruton[31] and Johnston et al.[32,33] demonstrated transpeptidation in kinetically controlled reactions. During the hydrolysis of Bz-Gly-NH_2 by

11

papain in the presence of $^{15}NH_3$, incorporation of ^{15}N in the recovered Bz-Gly-NH_2 was found in amounts higher than accountable by reversal of hydrolysis.[31] Hydroxamic acids were synthesized from N-protected amino acid amides in the presence of hydroxylamine by papain, a synthesis that could not be brought about in appreciable amounts using N-protected amino acids and hydroxylamine[32]. Chymotrypsin was used[33] to transpeptidize Bz-Tyr-Gly-NH_2 and Bz-Tyr-NH_2 in the presence of ^{15}N-labelled Gly-NH_2 and $^{15}NH_3$, respectively. Whereas transpeptidation could be demonstrated in the first case, only slight amounts of ammonia were exchanged in Bz-Tyr-NH_2. Bz-Tyr-Gly-NH_2 was later obtained[34] by transpeptidation of Bz-Ty-NH_2 in the presence of Gly-NH_2, pointing at ammonia as the cause of the failure in the transpeptidation reaction, most likely due to its high pK. A definition of transpeptidation and transamidation reactions was put forward[32], viz. replacement reactions in which one participant in a peptide or amide bond is replaced by another, closely related, molecular species. Although the mechanism proposed, featuring two nitrogen atoms attached to the carbon atom of the carbonyl group, no longer holds true, the definition fits very well with the mechanism for serine and thiol proteases, equations (xiv) and (xv).

Brenner et al.[35] treated L,D-methionine esters with chymotrypsin and obtained precipitates consisting of the L-forms of Met-Met and Met-Met-Met under concomitant formation of free methionine, in a kinetically controlled peptide synthesis with partial protection against hydrolysis of the peptides in the solid phase. Yields of peptides were about 30% of the L-methionine esters.

The newer studies aiming at exploiting the proteases for preparative purposes are clearly classified in kinetically and thermodynamically controlled syntheses. In the kinetically controlled synthesis, in its most commonly used form, the carboxyl component, as an alkyl ester, reacts in aqueous solution at about pH 9.5 with a serine (or thiol) protease yielding the acyl-enzyme, equation (xiv). High pH favours the esterolytic action of the serine proteases over the peptidolytic action. In the subsequent reaction, water and amino components compete for the acyl-enzyme yielding the carboxyl component as the free acid and the desired peptide, respectively, equation (xv). With careful control of reaction conditions and time the desired peptide can be obtained in fair yields. The kinetically controlled peptide synthesis has been developed by Breddam, Johansen and Widmer using carboxy-peptidase Y for stepwise peptide chain elongation[36-40].

In the thermodynamically controlled peptide syntheses high concentrations of reactants, especially of the least expensive one, are used to displace the equilibrium towards syntheses. Two methods of increasing yields dominate: precipitation of the product from solution and addition of organic solvents. If the protecting groups of the reactants are selected among the aromatic and larger aliphatic groups, precipitation of the product from aqueous solution will drive equation (vi) to the right. Using such principles Oka and Morihara synthesized a number of smaller peptides using trypsin[41], chymotrypsin[42], thermolysin[43] and subtilisin, papain and pepsin[44].

The other obvious way to exploit the law of mass action, namely by reducing the activity of water by adding an organic co-solvent, was first introduced by Ingalls *et al.* in the synthesis of *N*-acetyltyrosine ethyl ester[45] in a medium containing a high concentration of ethanol using chymotrypsin and subtilisin Carlsberg, (xvii):

(xvii) $CH_3CO\text{-}Tyr\text{-}OH + C_2H_5OH \rightleftharpoons CH_3CO\text{-}Tyr\text{-}OC_2H_5 + H_2O$

It was found that the activity of both free and immobilized chymotrypsin was better preserved if polyvalent alcohols like glycerol and ethylene glycol were present in the mixture together with ethanol. Alcohols are not excluded as co-solvents when the desired product is a peptide, as a primary amine is usually a much better nucleophile than an aliphatic alcohol in the reaction with the acyl-enzyme. However, ester formation may complicate peptide bond synthesis when reactions are performed in alcohols; see Chapter 4.

For newer reviews on the application of enzymes in the synthesis of peptide bonds, see Laskowski[46] and Chaiken *et al.*[47], Fruton[48] and Jakubke *et al.*[49].

The theory of the effect of organic co-solvents put forward by Homandberg *et al.* in 1978[14] initiated the insulin transubstantiation studies using thermodynamically controlled synthesis. In most relevant literature the activity of water has been equalled to unity. As the activity of water is reduced by addition of substantial amounts of organic solvents, the molar concentration of water has been included in the assessment of the apparent equilibrium constants in the present treatise. Activity coefficients have, due to lack of data, been equalled to unity throughout. The experimentally found variations in the apparent equilibrium constants between solvents reflect variations in activity coefficients as well as variations of the ionization term, equation (vii).

3. FROM PORCINE TO HUMAN INSULIN USING TRYPSIN

The primary structure of human insulin was published by Nicol and Smith in 1960[50], Figure 1. The high degree of identity to the already known structure of porcine insulin published by Brown *et al.* in 1955[51] caused much speculation of how to convert porcine insulin to human insulin, the only difference being the C-terminal residue of the B-chain, position B 30, where porcine insulin features an alanine, human insulin a threonine residue. That the neighbouring residue, B29, is a lysine suggested the possible usefulness of trypsin with its specificity for basic residues, a complication being that residue B22 is an arginine, another site for tryptic attack.

One such unpublished speculation by Markussen from 1968 is shown schematically in Figure 2. One further objection to the strategy lies in step 1, the tertiary butylation of the carboxyl groups without destruction of the insulin molecule. A strategy where use is made of tryptic hydrolysis at Arg^{B22} was published by Ruttenberg in 1972[52], see Figure 3. One weak point of this strategy was pointed out by König and Volk[53], namely that the Asn^{A21}-OMe residue upon saponification forms a succinimide that very slowly opens to a mixture of α- and β-asparagine residues. The second attempt to make semisynthetic human insulin where use is made of trypsin hydrolysis at

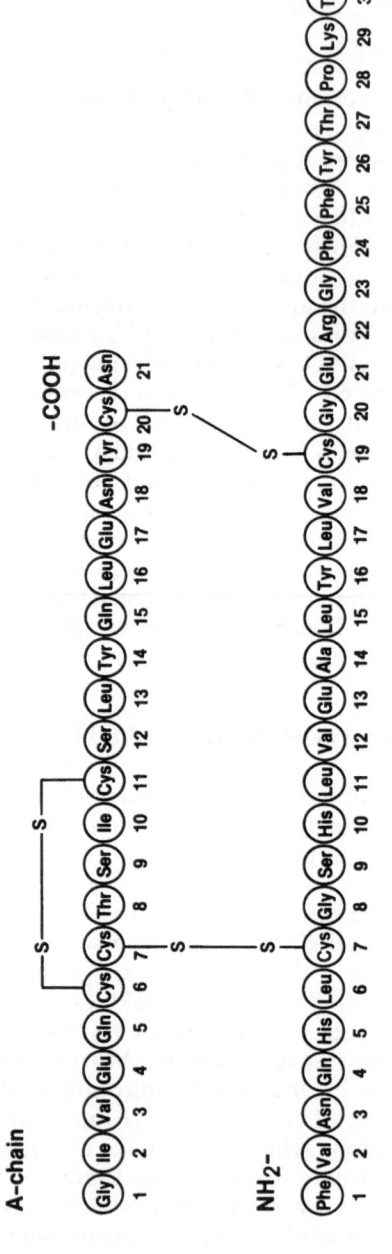

Figure 1 Structure of human insulin[50].

Porcine insulin

Tertiary butylation of six carboxylic acid residues in acidic, anhydrous medium.

$\left[\text{Glu}^{\text{A4, A17, B13, B21}} (\text{-OBu}^t) \right]_4$, $\text{Asn}^{\text{A21}}\text{-OBu}^t$, $\text{Ala}^{\text{B30}}\text{-OBu}^t$ porcine insulin

Cleavage by trypsin, release of Ala-OBu^t.

$\left[\text{Glu}^{\text{A4, A17, B13, B21}} (\text{-OBu}^t) \right]_4$, $\text{Asn}^{\text{A21}}\text{-OBu}^t$, des-(B30) insulin

Acylation by Boc–azide

Boc-α-Gly$^{\text{A1}}$, Boc-α-Phe$^{\text{B1}}$, Boc-ε-Lys$^{\text{B29}}$, $\left[\text{Glu}^{\text{A4, A17, B13, B21}} \right.$ $\left. (\text{-OBu}^t) \right]_4$, $\text{Asn}^{\text{A21}}\text{-OBu}^t$, des-(B30) insulin

Coupling to L-Thr-OBu^t using DCC

Boc-α-Gly$^{\text{A1}}$, Boc-α-Phe$^{\text{B1}}$, Boc-ε-Lys$^{\text{B29}}$, $\left[\text{Glu}^{\text{A4, A17, B13, B21}} \right.$ $\left. (\text{-OBu}^t) \right]_4$, $\text{Asn}^{\text{A21}}\text{-OBu}^t$, $\text{Thr}^{\text{B30}}\text{-OBu}^t$ human insulin

Deprotection by anhydrous TFA

Human insulin

Figure 2 Strategy for semisynthetic conversion of porcine insulin to human insulin (Markussen 1968, unpublished)

Arg$^{\text{B22}}$ was the work of Obermeier and Geiger[54]. The strategy (see Figure 4) is similar to that of Ruttenberg, but the coupling of the synthetic octapeptide B(23–30) to (Boc)$_2$A1,B1-desoctapeptide-(B23–B30) insulin was carried out with no protection of the five carboxyl groups of Glu$^{\text{A4}}$, Glu$^{\text{A17}}$, Asn$^{\text{A21}}$, Glu$^{\text{B13}}$ and Glu$^{\text{B21}}$. Since the coupling took place preferentially at the carboxyl group of Arg$^{\text{B22}}$ rather than at the other five, the synthesis of human insulin by this ambiguous route was achieved in a yield of about 10%, after extensive chromatography.

In the hitherto mentioned proposals use has been made only of the hydrolytic action of trypsin to split at Arg$^{\text{B22}}$ or Lys$^{\text{B29}}$. The first proposal to use trypsin or carboxypeptidase A to transpeptidize porcine insulin to human insulin was a patent by Bodanszky and Fried[55] in 1966 (xviii):

$$\text{(xviii)} \qquad \text{PI} + \text{Thr} \xrightarrow{\text{carboxypeptidase A or trypsin}} \text{HI} + \text{Ala}$$

Since the large excess of threonine was present as the free amino acid, its amino group was largely protonated as zwitterion at pH 7.8 where the

15

Porcine insulin

↓ **Diazomethane, pH 4.6**

$\left[\text{Glu}^{\text{A4, A17, B13, B21}}(\text{-OMe}) \right]_4$, Asn$^{\text{A21}}$-OMe, Ala$^{\text{B30}}$-OMe

porcine insulin

↓ **Cleavage by trypsin**

$\left[\text{Glu}^{\text{A4, A17, B13, B21}}(\text{-OMe}) \right]_4$, Asn$^{\text{A21}}$-OMe, desoctapeptide –

(B23–B30) insulin

↓ **Acylation by Boc-azide**

Boc-α-Gly$^{\text{A1}}$, Boc-α-Phe$^{\text{B1}}$, $\left[\text{Glu}^{\text{A4, A17, B13, B21}}(\text{-OMe}) \right]_4$,

Asn$^{\text{A21}}$-OMe desoctapeptide-(B23–B30) insulin

↓ **Coupling to Boc-ε-Lys$^{\text{B29}}$, Thr$^{\text{B30}}$-OMe, B(23-30) octapeptide using DCC/HOSu**

Boc-α-Gly$^{\text{A1}}$, Boc-α-Phe$^{\text{B1}}$, Boc-ε-Lys$^{\text{B29}}$, $\Big[\text{Glu}^{\text{A4, A17, B13, B21}}$

$(\text{-OMe}) \Big]_4$, Asn$^{\text{A21}}$-OMe, Thr$^{\text{B30}}$-OMe human insulin

↓ **Deprotection by anhydrous TFA**

$\left[\text{Glu}^{\text{A4, A17, B13, B21}}(\text{-OMe}) \right]_4$, Asn$^{\text{A21}}$-OMe, Thr$^{\text{B30}}$-OMe human insulin

↓ **Alkaline hydrolysis**

↓

Human insulin

Figure 3 Strategy for semisynthetic conversion of porcine insulin to human insulin, Ruttenberg[52]

reactions were carried out, reducing its reactivity in the deacylation by aminolysis, equation (xv). The author has repeated example 2 of the patent using trypsin in aqueous solution. It was found from the amino acid composition of the product that its composition was: unconverted PI: 32%; DAI: 8%; desoctapeptide-(B23–B30) insulin: 60%. The yield of human insulin could, by HPLC of the product, be estimated to amount to less than 1% of the product.

Porcine insulin

Cleavage by trypsin

desoctapeptide-(B23–B30) insulin

Acylation by Boc-OSu

Boc-α-Gly^{A1}, Boc-α-Phe^{B1}, desoctapeptide-(B23–B30) insulin

Coupling to Tyr^{B26}(Bu^t), Lys^{B29}(Boc), Thr^{B30}(Bu^t)-OBu^t
octapeptide-(B23–B30) using DCC/HOBt

Boc-α-Gly^{A1}, Boc-α-Phe^{B1}, Tyr^{B26}(Bu^t), Lys^{B29}(Boc),
Thr^{B30}(Bu^t)-OBu^t human insulin

Deprotection by anhydrous TFA

Human insulin

Figure 4 Semisynthesis of human insulin, Obermeier and Geiger[54]

Inouye *et al.* in 1979[56] were first in insulin chemistry to apply the effect of organic solvents on the reversal of peptide bond hydrolysis, equation (xi), published in 1978[13,14]. They coupled (Boc)$_2$-desoctapeptide-(B23–B30) insulin to synthetic Gly-Phe-Phe-Tyr-Thr-Pro-Lys(Boc)-Thr(Bu^t)-OBu^t by trypsin in a 1:1 mixture of DMF and an aqueous Tris buffer, apparent pH 6.5. With concentrations of Boc$_2$-DOI and protected octapeptide of 16.3 and 163 mM, respectively, a yield of 58% of protected insulin was found after 20 h at 37° C.

Des(Ala^{B30}) porcine insulin (DAI) became easily available in 1978 thanks to the method developed by Schmitt and Gattner[57]. They found that digestion of porcine insulin with carboxypeptidase A in an ammonium hydrogen carbonate buffer resulted specifically in release of Ala^{B30}, without release of Asn^{A21}, whereas in a Tris buffer both C-terminals were cleaved off. As B29 is a lysine and A20 is a half cystine no further cleavage occurs with carboxypeptidase A as shown by Slobin and Carpenter[58].

First to make use of DAI in synthesis of human insulin were Morihara *et al.*[59]. The guanidino group of Arg^{B22} of DAI thus prepared was temporarily protected by the Dhch-group to avoid tryptic cleavage. After coupling of Arg(Dhch)^{B22}-DAI to Thr-OBu^t by trypsin in DMF/ethanol/water (about 30/30/40) at an apparent pH of 6.5 at 38°C overnight, the protecting groups were removed with 1 M hydroxylamine (Dhch) and TFA (OBu^t). The overall yield was estimated as 50%.

Eventually Morihara et al.[60] ventured a coupling in DMF/ethanol/water of DAI with Thr-OBu^t by trypsin without side-chain protection of Arg^{B22}. 'To our surprise, there was no splitting of the Arg(B22)–Gly(B23) bond in DAI or the product; this was expected to be a problem, and has previously been thought to occur through the hydrolytic activity of trypsin[3].' The results of tryptic action on insulin causing cleavages at Arg^{B22} and Lys^{B29} were described by Wang and Carpenter[61]. As the success of this simple strategy was a surprise to the experts, patents were granted[62]. The conditions for the coupling reaction were: solvent DMF/ethanol/water about 30/30/40. Trypsin 0.1 mM; DAI 10 mM; Thr-OBu^t 0.5 M; Tris 0.2 M. Apparent pH 6.5, presumably adjusted with acetic acid? Reaction 20 h at 37°C. The yield of HI-OBu^t was determined by RP-HPLC to be 73%, HI-OBu^t being designated 'b' in the chromatogram. Morihara et al.[60] designated the first large peak of the chromatogram 'a' as being due to unreacted DAI, not realizing that DOI-Thr-OBu^t coelutes with DAI on columns of Nucleosil $5C_{18}$ at acid pH. A peak not commented on, eluting between 'a' and 'b' and amounting to about 10% of the total, could be DOI-Thr(Bu^t)-OBu^t, arising from Thr(Bu^t)-OBu^t, a very likely contaminant in Thr-OBu^t. The corresponding insulin, HI(Bu^t)-OBu^t was not revealed, since it requires a gradient in acetonitrile to about 38% in order to emerge from the column. Despite the arguable conclusion that there was no splitting at the Arg(B22)–Gly(B23) bond, the authors had demonstrated that synthesis without arginine side-chain protection is possible. Based on the present knowledge the yield can be considered as a rate and equilibrium controlled result of six reactions (xix, xx, xxi, xxii, xxiii and xxiv):

(xix)   Coupling: $DAI + Thr\text{-}OBu^t \rightleftharpoons HI\text{-}OBu^t + H_2O$

(xx)   Transpeptidation: $DAI + Thr\text{-}OBu^t \rightarrow DOI\text{-}Thr\text{-}OBu^t + B(23\text{-}29)$

(xxi)   Transpeptidation: $HI\text{-}OBu^t + Thr\text{-}OBu^t \rightarrow DOI\text{-}Thr\text{-}OBu^t$
$+ B(23\text{-}30)OBu^t$

(xxii) Denaturation: $Trypsin \xrightarrow{f(temp.,[H_2O])} inactive\ trypsin$

(xxiii) Hydrolysis: $DAI + H_2O \rightarrow DOI + B(23\text{-}29)$

(xxiv) Hydrolysis: $HI\text{-}OBu^t + H_2O \rightarrow DOI + B(23\text{-}30)\text{-}OBu^t$

Since the coupling reaction (xix) is faster than the transpeptidation reactions (xx) and (xxi) and trypsin is degraded adequately fast in an aqueous–organic medium at 37°C, a fair yield was obtained. The equilibrium, equation (xix), is actually displaced far more favourably towards synthesis than the 27/73 ratio between the peaks 'a' and 'b' of the chromatogram seems to indicate; possibly only a small percentage of peak 'a' represents unreacted DAI. The final step from HI-OBu^t to HI was accomplished by TFA.

Shortly after Gattner et al.[63] presented a very similar synthesis (xxv):

(xxv) $DAI + Thr\text{-}OMe \rightleftharpoons HI\text{-}OMe + H_2O$

The conditions for the coupling reaction were: DMF/water 6/4; buffer 0.08 M pyridinium acetate; DAI 8.4 mM; Thr-OMe,HCl 0.42 M; trypsin: three additions, each 0.07 mM at 0, 2 and 6 h. Reaction at 38°C at an apparent pH of 6.5 for 20 h. The ratio between DAI and HI-OMe was found to be 33/67. Neither DOI-Thr-OMe nor DOI are to be seen in the HPLC chromatogram; both components that emerge much earlier than DAI on RP-HPLC. The yield of coupling of 67% would have been higher if Thr-OMe had not been introduced as the hydrochloride salt, the 0.08 M pyridinium acetate being unable to neutralize the HCl of 0.42 M Thr-OMe,HCl, pyridine being a weaker base than Thr-OMe (xxvi):

(xxvi)   Thr-OMe,HCl + pyridine ← pyridine,HCl + Thr-OMe

As it is the concentration of Thr-OMe with an unprotonated amino group that displaces equation (xxv) towards peptide bond synthesis, hydrochlorides should be avoided, unless they are neutralized with an appropriately strong base. The conversion of HI-OMe to HI in this synthesis disclosed a surprisingly mild hydrolysis of the threonine methyl ester of HI-OMe. The saponification was completed after 3 days at room temperature at pH 9.5. Once again, surprise was expressed that no peptide bond cleavage had taken place at Arg^{B22} in this mixture of water and organic solvents. Coletti-Previora et al.[64] had demonstrated earlier that esterolytic action of trypsin was retained in 75% dioxan, 25% formamide and 37% 2-chloroethanol, whereas the amidolytic action was abolished in all three mixtures. Hence, the stability against hydrolysis at Arg^{B22}-Gly^{B23} was not totally unpredictable.

It was therefore equally surprising when Markussen[65] in 1980 showed that peptide bond cleavage could in fact be conducted in such media between Lys^{B29} and Ala^{B30} by trypsin in a transpeptidation reaction (xxvii):

(xxvii)   Porcine insulin + Thr-OR → HI-OR + Ala

This was the first report on transpeptidation in aqueous–organic media, but apparently the time was ripe for the idea, because within the 18 months between filing and divulgence of the patent application, three other groups made the same invention[66-68]. The detailed study of this reaction is the subject of Chapters 4 and 6. Porcine proinsulin, a contaminant of crude, crystallized porcine insulin, was likewise shown to be convertible to HI-OMe[65].

Markussen and Schaumburg made an attempt to examine whether a major part of the HI-OMe synthesized by transpeptidation had been hydrolysed to DAI and coupled again to HI-OMe, twice passing the same intermediate, the acyl-enzyme[69]. $H_2^{17}O$ was present in the reaction medium, and the incorporation of ^{17}O in the product, equation (xxviii), was studied by NMR:

$$\text{(xxviii) Porcine insulin + trypsin } \xrightarrow{-\text{Ala}} \text{ DAI-trypsin} \begin{cases} \pm H_2^{17}O \longrightarrow DAI(^{17}O\text{-labelled}) \\ \pm \text{Thr-OMe} \longrightarrow HI\text{-OMe}(^{17}O?) \end{cases}$$

19

Only if hydrolysis to DAI takes place is ^{17}O incorporated in the final product, in the carbonyl oxygen of Lys^{B29}. No such labelling was demonstrated, the conclusion being that DAI is not an intermediate in transpeptidation of porcine insulin to human insulin methyl ester under the conditions specified. This result is inconsistent with the kinetics of the conversion of DAI to HI-OMe in conjunction with the ratio between DAI and HI-OMe in equilibrium, as will be discussed in Chapter 6.

Markussen and Vølund studied the kinetics of transpeptidation and coupling of porcine insulin and DAI, respectively, with Thr-OMe and Thr(Bu^t)-OBu^t at a set of conditions where trypsin is stable[70,71]. It was found that coupling proceeds faster than transpeptidation. Coupling with Thr-OMe proceeds faster than with Thr(Bu^t)-OBu^t but transpeptidation occurs at a higher rate with Thr(Bu^t)-OBu^t than with Thr-OMe. It was concluded that Thr-OMe inhibits transpeptidation but not coupling. Yields of HI-OMe and of HI(Bu^t)-OBu^t eventually became similar, about 96%. The association between porcine insulin and trypsin was found to be so weak in the medium that K_m values could be estimated only as being larger than 0.1 M.

The reaction progress curves using the above mentioned conditions were simulated by numerical integration of the rate equations using the fourth-order Runge–Kutta method, and fitting the constants by trial and error[71]. In the model the inhibitory effect of Thr-OMe on the transpeptidation reaction was assumed to occur in the acyl-enzyme forming step by preferential binding of Thr-OMe to His^{46} at the active site of trypsin, leading to different rate constants for this step when using either Thr-OMe or Thr(Bu^t)-OBu^t. In the simpler model, presented in Chapter 6, this action of Thr-OMe is treated as a competitive inhibition of the association between insulin and trypsin. By binding of Thr-OMe to subsite S_1' of trypsin, association with porcine insulin and human insulin esters is inhibited, whereas association with des-(B30) insulin is unaffected. Both models can be fitted equally well to experimental data, but in the new model rate constants for covalent reactions become independent of the threonine ester in the medium.

The organic solvent can also be the reactant threonine ester used in large excess; Obermeier and Seipke thus used Thr(Bu^t)-OBu^t, added as the acetate salt and amounting to about 50% of the total (w/w), as the organic solvent[66,72]. Yields as high as 85% were reported. Formation of DOI was suppressed by adding acetic acid to 'pH 4.5' as measured with a glass electrode in the mixture. In an experiment[72] with equimolar amounts of Thr-OMe and Thr(Bu^t)-OBu^t the two human esters were synthesized with 'conversion rates' of HI-OMe = 6% and HI(Bu^t)-OBu^t = 50%. Whatever the meaning of '%', rate or yield, the result is different from what was found in another medium[70] where k(HI-OMe)/k(HI(Bu^t)-OBu^t) was 6/1 and the yield ratio HI-OMe/HI(Bu^t)-OBu^t was 52/44 at equilibrium.

Jonczyk and Gattner[68,73] converted porcine insulin to HI-OBu^t in Tris/HCl buffers between 'pH' 5.8 and 9.2 in water/DMF and found a dynamic optimum for HI-OMe synthesis using 67% (v/v) DMF, 'pH' 6.6 and 23°C, the 'pH' being defined as the reading of a glass electrode in the medium. They found that formation of DOI decreased at lower 'pH' values, causing the pH-optimum to move to 'pH' 5.8 as the reaction time was increased to 19 h. Very little synthesis was found at 'pH' 6.7 in 80%(v/v) DMF at 23°C, a result which is probably due to enzyme destruction, as excellent yields were obtained in only 20% H_2O in DMAC at 12°C[65]. An interesting finding was that phosphate buffers to a large extent suppress the side-reaction at Arg^{B22}, possibly by formation of complexes with the guanidino group[73].

Offord and Rose[74] and Rose et al.[75] converted porcine insulin to HI(Bu^t)-OBu^t in high yields (99%) in 2 h at 37°C in mixtures of BD, DMSO and water, containing down to about 5% water and using BD as the predominant organic solvent. The optimal pH was found to be 5.3–5.6 using indicator paper. In BD trypsin retained activity down to about 3% water even at 37°C. However, as shown in Chapter 4, BD is not by itself able to induce specificity for transpeptidation at Lys^{B29} rather than at Arg^{B22}. Substitution cf BD with glycerol markedly reduced the yields[75].

Rose et al.[76] studied the reaction (xxix):

$$\text{(xxix) Porcine insulin + trypsin} \xrightarrow{-\text{Ala}} \text{DAI-trypsin} \begin{cases} \pm \text{ DAI } (^{18}\text{O labelled}) \\ \pm \text{ H}_2{}^{18}\text{O} \\ \pm \text{ Thr(Bu}^t)\text{-OBu}^t \\ \text{HI(Bu}^t)\text{-OBu}^t(^{18}\text{O}) \end{cases}$$

in a medium containing $H_2{}^{18}O$ (6%), BD (about 70%), acetic acid (4%) and Thr(Bu^t)-OBu^t (about 20%). The incorporation of ^{18}O in human insulin was studied by mass-spectrometry of the C-terminal tetrapeptide of the B-chain, Thr-Pro-Lys-Thr, obtained by successive digestions with pepsin and leucine aminopeptidase. Rapid incorporation of ^{18}O was found in Lys^{B29} carbonyl, equilibrating at 75% ^{18}O and 25% ^{16}O which apparently was the ratio between $H_2{}^{18}O$ and $H_2{}^{16}O$ in the solution. The result is contradictory to the study using $H_2{}^{17}O$ and NMR-spectroscopy[69] in another medium, where no incorporation was found; see Chapter 6 where the validity of the ^{17}O-NMR study is questioned.

4. ALTERNATIVE PROTEASES

Breddam et al.[77,78] investigated the use of carboxypeptidase Y from yeast to transpeptidize porcine insulin to human insulin in aqueous solution at pH 9.5 using Thr-NH_2 as amino component. A series of reactions occur, e.g. (xxx, xxxi, xxxii, xxxiii and xxxiv):

(xxx)   Porcine insulin + Thr-NH_2 → HI-NH_2 + Ala

(xxxi)   HI-NH_2 + Thr-NH_2 → HI-Thr-NH_2 + NH_3

(xxxii)   HI-Thr-NH_2 → HI + Thr-NH_2

(xxxiii)   HI-NH_2 → DAI + Thr-NH_2

(xxxiv)   HI-NH_2 → HI + NH_3

Although human insulin is formed in a single-step reaction in water this reaction has not been exploited in human insulin production as there are at present no means to separate PI, HI and DAI preparatively. Yields of 30% human insulin were reported isolating HI-Thr-NH$_2$ and HI-NH$_2$ as intermediates and then carrying out the reaction (xxxiv) at pH 10, where carboxypeptidase Y has no peptidase activity. Breddam and Johansen improved the yields when carboxypeptidase Y chemically modified in the active site with methyl mercuric iodide was used both for the transpeptidation reaction (xxx) in 1 M urea at pH 8 and for the deamidation reaction (xxxiv) at pH 10[79,80].

Morihara et al.[81] investigated the use of *Achromobacter lyticus* protease in the coupling reaction (xix), in which earlier they had used trypsin[60]. The *A. lyticus* protease is more specific than trypsin, in that it only cleaves the carboxylic bonds of lysine residues as shown by Masaki et al.[82]. The yields (60–80%) appear to be similar using either the *A. lyticus* protease or trypsin. The *A. lyticus* protease also served to prepare the DAI from porcine insulin by initial hydrolysis in aqueous solution.

Muneyuki et al.[83] immobilized *A. lyticus* protease to an aminopropyl-silica gel via a poly-glutamyl linker. In repeated couplings this preparation yielded about 70% HI-OBu^t, equation (xix), using only 28% 'solvent' (DMF/ethanol: 1/1) at pH 6.5 at 37°C, 5 mM DAI and 0.8 M Thr-OBu^t, a surprisingly high degree of synthesis at such high concentration of water, cf. equations (i, ii and iii). Morihara and Oka[84] compared the efficacy of *A. lyticus* protease and trypsin in the coupling reaction (xix) and found *A. lyticus* to have a turnover number about 10 times that of trypsin. They also compared coupling, reaction (xix), and transpeptidation, reaction (xxvii), in 0.8 M Thr-OBu^t, 1.5 M acetic acid, 31% H$_2$O, 43% ethanol/DMF (1/1), 'pH' $\sim$ 5.5, using the *A. lyticus* protease, and found that transpeptidation requires about 100 times more enzyme to proceed at a comparable rate. They conclude that since much enzyme is required for transpeptidation and since the specific activity decreases as a result of immobilization to the carrier, the best combination using immobilized enzyme is coupling with immobilized *A. lyticus*. However, Soejima et al.[85] from the company supplying the *A. lyticus* protease (Wako) obtained fair yields transpeptidizing porcine insulin to HI-OBu^t using immobilized 'lysine specific protease', i.e. *A. lyticus* protease I.

Examples of the use of the *A. lyticus* protease to transpeptidize single-chain insulin precursors resistant to reaction will be dealt with in Chapter 6.

5. SINGLE-CHAIN INSULINS

In a trypsin catalysed, intramolecular transpeptidation Markussen et al.[86] converted porcine insulin to single-chain des-(B30) insulin (SCI) in a medium devoid of primary amino groups except those of the insulin molecule, equation (xxxv):

(xxxv)   Porcine insulin → SCI + Ala

A yield of 13% was achieved in a buffer equimolar in acetic acid and N-methyl morpholine, the solvent being about 21% water in DMAC. As this molecule, SCI, can be reduced and reoxidized with better recovery than porcine proinsulin[87] it renders itself a candidate for a precursor molecule in the biosynthesis of insulin[88]. The transpeptidation of three single-chain precursor molecules, SCI = B(1–29)-A(1–21) insulin, B(1–29)-Ala-Ala-Lys-A(1–21) insulin and B(1–29)-Ser-Lys-A(1–21) insulin is the topic of Chapter 5, whereas the transpeptidation of the single-chain porcine proinsulin molecule is dealt with in Chapter 4.

6. PREPARATION OF HUMAN INSULIN

After the conversion reaction the enzyme must be removed or inactivated under conditions that are harmless to the synthesized human insulin ester. Using immobilized enzymes this step is a simple filtration. Using soluble enzymes the most commonly used method is a gel filtration in 1 M acetic acid in which trypsin is inactive. Subsequently, an anion exchange chromatography is introduced to separate HI-OR from DAI, porcine insulin and DOI-Thr-OR. Finally the ester group of HI-OR is cleaved by acidolysis (-OBu^t) or by hydrolysis (-OMe). Selected preparative procedures for such operations have been published[89].

7. DERIVATIVES OF HUMAN INSULIN

D-allo-threonine^{B30}-OMe human insulin was synthesized in fair yields from porcine insulin and D-allo-Thr-OMe by trypsin, using the reaction conditions of the kinetic studies in Chapter 6 (Lundt and Markussen, 1980, unpublished). This means that L-configuration is not an absolute requirement for binding to the S_1' site of trypsin at the conditions that bring about peptide bond synthesis.

Inouye et al.[90] described couplings of (Boc)$_2$-DOI to B23–B30 octapeptides in which either Phe^{B24} or Phe^{B25} was substituted with D-Phe. Low yields were obtained with both octapeptides as compared to the all-L octapeptide, meaning that subsites S_2' and S_3' recognize the substrate configuration to some extent.

Obermeier and Seipke[72] reported rates (probably yields, in %) of conversion of porcine insulin to various B30-substituted insulin esters. The 'rate' increased through the series:

$$Gly\text{-}OBu^t = Ala\text{-}OBu^t < Ser(Bu^t)\text{-}OBu^t < Thr\text{-}OMe$$

$$< Phe\text{-}OBu^t < Val\text{-}OBu^t$$

$$= Thr(Bu^t)\text{-}OBu^t < Leu\text{-}OBu^t$$

There is no obvious relationship between structure and 'rate'. Interestingly, the leaving amino acid is of importance to the 'rate', e.g. the 'rate' of Ala^{B30}-OBu^t insulin is much lower when human insulin is the substrate (5%) than when porcine insulin is the substrate (25%). In couplings between DAI and various amino acid esters and amides Gattner et al.[91] found increasing yields through the series:

$$Ala\text{-}OBu^t < Ala\text{-}NH_2 < Ala\text{-}OMe < Tyr\text{-}OMe < Thr\text{-}NH_2$$

$$< Thr\text{-}OMe < Glu\text{-}(OMe)_2$$

The combined results seem to indicate that Ala-OBu^t is a poor amino component in both transpeptidation and coupling, unless it was applied coincidentally as the hydrochloride by both groups of investigators.

2
Materials and methods

1. THE ENZYMATIC CONVERSION REACTION, SCALE AND EXECUTION

The coupling and transpeptidation reactions were carried out in stoppered, 5 ml test tubes (10 × 100 mm). In a typical experiment 20 mg of insulin component was weighed out in the test tube and dissolved in 100 μl of an aqueous solution of acetic acid, to which was added 200 μl of 2 M threonine ester dissolved in the organic solvent to be examined. In most cases the ester was applied as the free base. Varying the concentration of acetic acid results in buffers either of the ammonium/amino type (H^+-Thr-OR/Thr-OR) or of the carboxylic acid/carboxylate type (CH_3COOH/CH_3COO^-). As the dissociation of carboxylic acids is suppressed by addition of organic solvents[11,12,14], whereas ammonium acids are virtually unaffected, the whole acid/base range of interest is covered by the reactant threonine ester and acetic acid and further addition of buffers (like Tris) has consequently been omitted. The pK for Thr-OMe in water was found to be 6.8 and for Thr(Bu^t)-OBu^t to be 7.2. The desired concentration of water was then adjusted by addition of 60 μl water and/or organic solvent. The solution was then thermostated at the reaction temperature. Finally 40 μl of a thermostated 5% (w/v) trypsin solution, viz. 2 mg of trypsin in 0.05 M aqueous calcium acetate, was added to start the reaction. It was noted that additions of solid trypsin to aqueous–organic mixtures effectively inactivated the trypsin. The total volume closely equals the sum of pipetted solutions, i.e. 400 μl, as contractions are counterbalanced by the volume of the dissolved insulin. Consequently the concentration of threonine ester could be set to 1 molar. Pipetting was found to be most precisely and reproducibly executed by an adjustable Eppendorf Vari Pipette (0–100 μl), rather than by constriction pipettes.

Using molecular weights of about 5900 for insulin compounds and 23 400 for trypsin, the concentrations are calculated to 8.4 mM and 0.22 mM, respectively. If corrections for a 5–10% water content of the two crystalline proteins are introduced the concentrations are about 8 mM and 0.2 mM.

The reaction was monitored by sampling 25 μl in thermostated constriction pipettes at appropriate intervals and precipitating the proteins in the sample by dilution in either 2 ml of acetone or in 2 ml of 15% (w/v) NaCl/0.11 M HCl in a 5 ml centrifuge tube. Both diluents quench the activity of trypsin. The precipitated proteins were isolated by centrifugation. Washings with 2 ml of acetone or 15% (w/v) NaCl/0.01 M HCl respectively, centrifugation and drying *in vacuo* completed the isolation. The dry samples were stored refrigerated until analysis. Using either method the threonine esters, the acetic acid and the organic solvent are discarded with the supernatants from the centrifugations. Each method, however, has slight advantages compared to the other. Human insulin esters of very hydrophobic character, like Thr^{B30}(Bu^t)-OBu^t insulin, are difficult to dissolve in small volumes of 1 M acetic acid for the subsequent analysis by HPLC in the presence of small amounts of NaCl and, in such cases, precipitation with acetone was preferred. Precipitation with NaCl results in a clearer HPLC chromatogram of insulin compounds since trypsin, its degradation products and octapeptide B(23-29)-Thr-OR are only to a limited extent salted out in 15% (w/v) NaCl. Such clearer chromatograms were preferred in kinetic studies, where interference from unknown degradation products eluting close to the position of the product, the human insulin ester, would result in estimation of falsely elevated rate constants. Salting out in NaCl/HCl results to a minor extent in deamidation of Asn^{A21}, resulting in compounds eluting just after the parent component. For a comparison of the two procedures cf. the HPLC

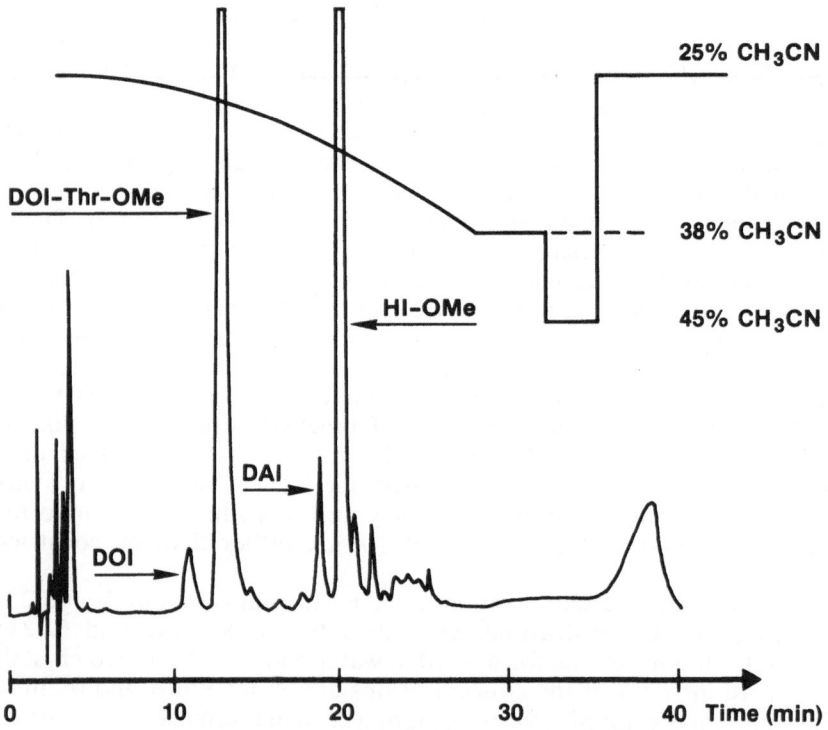

Figure 5 HPLC analysis of acetone precipitate of a reaction mixture from a conversion of porcine insulin to human insulin methyl ester, cf. Figure 6. Gradient elution

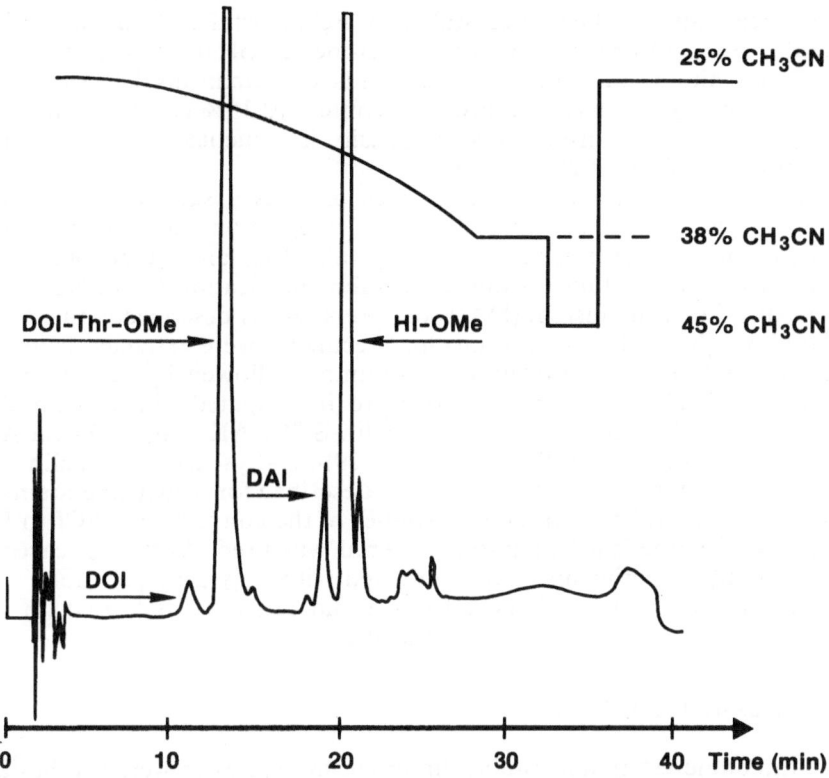

Figure 6 HPLC analysis of a NaCl/HCl precipitate of a reaction mixture from a conversion of porcine insulin to human insulin methyl ester. Sample taken in parallel to that of Figure 5. Gradient elution

chromatograms Figure 5 and Figure 6. Table 26 shows an experiment where the two methods of precipitation have been compared.

Two and multifactor experiments, with each factor at two to four levels, were set up in parallel in order to scan the space of parameters within a reasonable time, to detect any interplay and to make conclusions self-contained within the experiment. Up to 32 tubes were handled within a single plan. About 90 plans were conducted on transpeptidation of porcine insulin to human insulin esters, and about 50 on transpeptidation of single-chain insulin precursors to human insulin esters. Coupling reactions using DAI as substrate were studied as an integral part of the kinetics.

2. INSULIN COMPOUNDS

It was found quite early that impurities in porcine insulin such as proinsulin and intermediate products from the *in vivo* transformation of proinsulin to insulin were also converted to human insulin esters. Consequently a rather crude porcine insulin, the first crystal crop (FC), crystallized from a medium of 6 mM zinc, 50 mM citrate, 15% acetone at pH 6.1[92], was used for experiments aiming at optimizing the yields of human insulin ester. Such citrate insulin crystals having a low zinc content (0.35% corresponding to 2 Zn^{2+} per hexamer of insulin) dissolve easily in aqueous acetic acid up to concentrations of about 20% (w/v).

Porcine monocomponent insulin[93] was used as a substrate for kinetic studies in order to achieve improved HPLC integration due to reduced base line variations. Porcine insulin, first crystals (FC) and monocomponent quality (MC), were obtained from the Insulin Purification Plant, Novo.

Des-Ala^{B30} porcine insulin (DAI) was prepared as described earlier[89].

The biosynthetic single-chain insulin precursors were extracted from the fermentation broth by absorption to columns, followed by desorption as described earlier[88]. Three precursors were investigated, single-chain des-(B30) insulin (SCI) = B(1–29)-A(1–21) insulin, SCI-AAK = B(1–29)-Ala-Ala-Lys-A(1–21) insulin, and SCI-SK = B(1–29)-Ser-Lys-A(1–21) insulin. All three crystallized in zinc/citrate/ethanol as described for semisynthetic single-chain des-(B30) insulin[86]. In the first studies of the conversion of SCI to HI-OR, the semisynthetically prepared material was used. As it was scarce at the time, initial experiments were conducted with only 2 mg per tube.

Human insulin and its esters, HI-OMe and HI(Bu^t)-OBu^t, used for the kinetic studies, were prepared as described earlier[89].

3. THREONINE ESTERS

The L-threonine esters and D-allo-threonine methyl ester were synthesized at Novo in the Laboratory of Peptide Chemistry. They were prepared either as the free bases or as the hydroacetates. Hydrochlorides of threonine esters were deliberately avoided. Some physical constants of the L-threonine esters chosen for transpeptidation studies are compiled in Table 1. Thr-OMe and Thr(Bu^t)-OBu^t have been investigated most thoroughly because they are the most easily accessible examples of base- and acid-labile esters, respectively. Thr-OBu^t has the advantage of being more easily deprotected by TFA than Thr(Bu^t)-OBu^t, but Thr-OBu^t is far more difficult to prepare in good yields and with reasonable purity than Thr(Bu^t)-OBu^t. Impurities in the threonine esters were in no instance found to be related to reaction progress nor to cause trouble interpreting the chromatograms.

4. DEFINITION AND DETERMINATION OF WATER CONTENT

Homandberg et al.[14] estimated the activity of water by the vapour pressure above water/1,4-butanediol mixtures, ignoring the contribution from the organic solvent. In the lack of an electrode for measuring water activity, the water concentration has been used to denote this factor.

The concentration of water in reaction mixtures was determined by the Karl Fischer method in the Metrohm 652 KF coulometer equipment for microanalysis at the Novo Microanalytical Laboratory. The sample size amounts to 10 μl. Results are expressed in % water (w/v).

An expedient nominal percentage of water was calculated using the following approximations:

(a) The total volume equals the sum of the volumes of additions to constitute the mixture.

(b) The volume of the insulin compounds (usually 5% w/v) is not accounted for.

(c) The water content in mixtures of acetic acid and water equals $100(1 - [HOAc]/17.5)\%$.

The contractions when mixing solvents and the volume of dissolved insulin compounds counterbalance to some extent, and reasonable concordant values of nominal percentage of water and Karl Fischer analyses were found, the difference ranging from -0.6 to $+1.7\%$. Table 2 shows a comparison of nominal percentage of water and Karl Fischer analyses of patent examples[65] selected to cover a wide range of water concentrations. Karl Fischer water determinations were performed in selected experiments and data are included in Tables 37, 65, 66, 68, 72, and 75.

In the experiments where solids were used as organic solvent, the water content of solutions in water (8 M urea; 8, 10 and 12 M acetamide) was determined densitometrically. Acetic acid solutions and threonine ester solutions were made up from the solutions of urea and acetamide in water, calculating the water content in acetic acid solutions according to (c) and water content in threonine ester solutions by densitometry. Finally, approximations (a) and (b) were applied to calculate water content in the finished mixture.

As the water concentration is a tangible factor of importance for the yield, it has been chosen rather than the complementary percentage of organic solvent to characterize the mixtures. The insulin compounds and the threonine esters account for substantial amounts of the non-aqueous volume, typically 5% and 15%, respectively.

5. 'pH' MEASUREMENT IN MIXTURES OF WATER AND ORGANIC SOLVENTS

Readings on a pH meter using a glass electrode in mixtures of water and organic solvents can be a useful indicator of acidity as long as comparisons are made in the same medium only. Comparisons between media become virtually meaningless, as both the activity coefficients and the liquid-junction potentials are media dependent[94,95]. Michaelis and Mitzutani[11] defined the activity of hydrogen ions in ethanol–water mixtures as that of the aqueous solution, which has the same potential when measured with a hydrogen electrode. The authors realized that this definition is only practical when the liquid-junction potential can be ignored. Gutbezahl and Grunwald[96] calculated the liquid-junction potential between 80% ethanol in water and water to be 74.8 mV, corresponding to 1.26 pH units.

Douzou and Balny[97] provided a pragmatic definition of pH in aqueous–

organic mixtures, in which alternating solutions of buffers and colour indicators are used in a stepwise building up of a pH scale. As a basis between solvents a 10 mM solution of hydrochloric acid is used, assuming complete dissociation and using the Debye–Hückel equation to calculate the activity coefficient of the hydrogen ion in the actual media.

Despite these difficulties in defining pH in other solvents than water both Inouye et al.[56] and Jonczyk and Gattner[73] used glass electrodes to measure 'pH' in aqueous–organic solvent mixtures. Inappropriate use of the pH concept has even been applied in a patent claim to specify the inventive step (see ref. 66, claim 1): 'Process for the preparation of human insulin or its derivatives from pig insulin or its derivatives, characterized in that pig insulin or a derivative thereof is reacted at a pH value below its isoelectric point in the presence of trypsin... .' The reading of the glass electrode in water-organic solvent mixtures is thus being compared to the isoelectric point of insulin as determined in water!

The difference of glass electrode readings in buffered water-organic solvents and the pH values measured after a 100-fold dilution in water depends upon the solvent and the percentage of water. In Table 3 corresponding glass electrode readings and pH measurements after dilution are compared for seven selected examples from two patents.[65,66] Whereas there is agreement between measured pH and the calculated pH for buffered, aqueous solutions of weak acids using $pH = pK + \log(B/A)$, a positive difference is found between glass electrode reading and pH measured after a 100-fold dilution, ranging from 0.3 to 2 meter units. The difference increases with decreasing water content, and depends upon the type of organic solvent. In examples 6, 9 and 10 from the patent cited above[66], the organic solvent is the threonine ester itself, $Thr(Bu^t)$-OBu^t hydroacetate, accounting for about 50% of the volume. In this solvent the difference is smaller than in strong aprotic solvents like DMF, DMAC and HMPA for the same content of water.

Rose et al.[75] prefer to use indicator paper to reproduce acidity in reaction mixtures. Readings in organic media using indicator paper will to a large extent depend upon the type of indicator acid, viz. either of carboxylic/phenolic or of ammonium type.

The acidity will be coped with here by specifying the actual acid/base ratio (M/M) of the buffer system in the mixture. In the calculation of acid/base ratio acetic acid is by convention set to be a stronger acid than the ammonium form of threonine esters, although the dissociation of carboxylic acids is reduced in organic solvent and that of ammonium acids is affected to only a small degree. The apparent pKs of acetic acid, Thr-OMe and $Thr(Bu^t)$-OBu^t in 80% DMF were estimated at 8.1, 6.9 and 7.3, respectively, using a glass electrode.

Unless otherwise specified, $^+$H-Thr-OR/Thr-OR type buffers have been established from Thr-OR base and acetic acid.

6. ENZYMES

Twice crystallized porcine and bovine trypsin (EC 3.4.21.4) were obtained from the Department of Crystalline Enzymes, Novo. They were obtained as sterile preparations containing 5200 NF-units/mg (= USP-units/mg)[98], corresponding to 15 600 BAEE units/mg. As this represents a highly purified enzyme, molarities in solutions were estimated simply from enzyme weight × volume^{-1} × M_r^{-1}, using a molecular weight of porcine trypsin of 23 400[99], and making a 10% deduction from the weight due to crystal bound water.

The chymotrypsin activity of the twice crystallized (TC) porcine trypsin was < 50 NF-units/mg[98]. No side-reactions attributable to chymotrypsin activity were discovered. Treatment of trypsin with TPCK (L-(1-tosylamido-2-phenyl) ethyl chloromethyl ketone) according to Kostka and Carpenter[100] did not result in an improved specificity of the trypsin, as HPLC chromatograms of reaction mixtures using TPCK-treated trypsin and untreated trypsin appeared identical. Consequently TPCK treatment of the trypsin was eventually abandoned.

Porcine plasmin was obtained as a lyophilized preparation from the Department of Crystalline Enzymes, Novo. It contained 3.8 Novo units per mg corresponding to 125 Remmert and Cohn casein units/mg N[101]. The porcine plasminogen was activated either by trypsin or by urokinase. Both preparations of plasmin were studied.

Streptokinase (Sigma product No. S 3134, 4500 U/mg), Urokinase (Sigma U 6876, 2 U/mg) and Enterokinase (Sigma E 1256, 10 U/mg) were purchased from Sigma.

Lysyl endopeptidase from *Achromobacter lyticus* M497-1[82] was obtained from WAKO Pure Chemical Industries (Ltd.) Japan, in vials containing 10 AU (activity units) in a total of 7.4 mg of a lyophilized solid.

Porcine trypsin immobilized on glass beads (0.2 U/mg) and immobilized on Sephadex G-150 (1.5 U/mg) was obtained from the Enzyme Chemistry Laboratories, Novo. One trypsin unit (U) is the amount of trypsin that cleaves 1 μmole Bz-Arg-OEt (BAEE) per minute under specified conditions[102]. A crystalline porcine trypsin was analysed to 54 U/mg in this assay.

Succinylated trypsin was prepared according to a prescription obtained from the Enzyme Chemistry Laboratories, Novo: to 750 mg of trypsin dissolved in 150 ml 0.001 N HCl is added 450 mg succinic anhydride dissolved in 6 ml acetone at 0–5°C while stirring. The pH is adjusted to 7.0 and maintained at 7.0 during the reaction which takes 30 min. The reaction mixture is placed in a dialysis bag and dialysed against 10 litres distilled water for 24 hours, with a change of water after 8 hours. The dialysed material was lyophilized. Yield 630 mg. Activity = 37 U/mg. Degree of succinylation = 75% (ninhydrin test).

7. ANALYSIS BY DISC ELECTROPHORESIS

Disc electrophoresis in 7.5% polyacrylamide gels at pH 8.9 was carried out according to Davis[103] using the modifications described by Schlichtkrull *et al.*[93]. The samples, viz. 20 μl of each reaction mixture each containing 1 mg insulin compounds, were diluted with 200 μl of sample buffer (62 mM Tris, 60 mM HCl, 8 M urea) and 25 μl of the dilution was applied to the gels. The protein bands, stained with amidoschwarz, were evaluated visually using a graded set of standard gels with from 10 to 100 μg of porcine insulin in the insulin band. Thus the estimation of yields could be made with a precision better than $\pm 10\%$. The positions of the protein bands are shown in Figure 7.

The use of disc electrophoresis to evaluate reaction progress involves a number of drawbacks. Firstly, as indicated in Figure 7, porcine insulin and the by-product DOI-Thr-OR migrate to nearly the same position, making it difficult to assess whether a low yield of HI-OR is due to premature trypsin inactivation or lack of specificity. SCI also migrates to this position.[86] Secondly, the pH 8.9 in the running gel causes partial saponification of the human insulin ester when it is HI-OMe, resulting in a stained smear between the insulin and the insulin ester bands. Thirdly, trypsin is not immediately inactivated in the 8 M urea buffer used for diluting the reaction mixtures, and partial reversal of the synthesis could take place. Harris[104] reported 75% inactivation of trypsin in 8 M urea at pH 7.8 within 2 minutes. However, as the analysis by disc electrophoresis was applied in the initial experiments only, where the temperature chosen was 37°C and the sampling time 24 hours or more, the trypsin was already thoroughly degraded during the reaction time, and complications due to trypsin activity during analysis were not noticed. Despite these drawbacks valuable results were obtained using this method during November and December, 1979, Markussen[65] examples 1 through 21. Examples of analysis by disc electrophoresis are shown in Figures 16, 18 and 19.

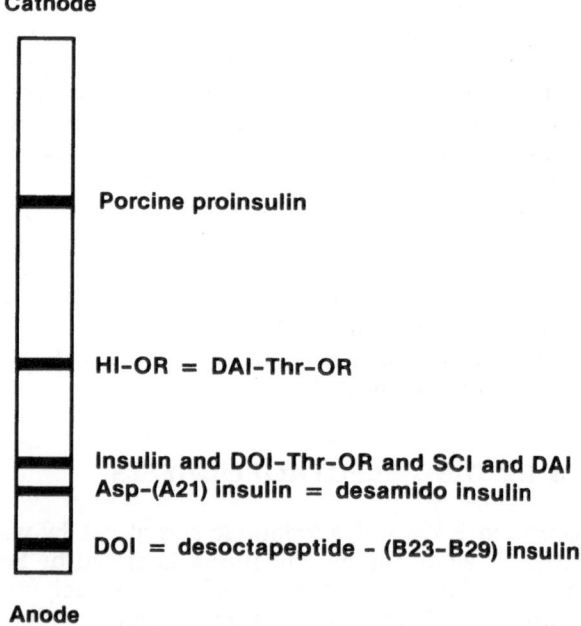

Figure 7 Positions of bands of insulin compounds present in reaction mixtures using disc electrophoresis at pH 8.9 in 7.5% polyacrylamide gel

8. ANALYSIS BY RP-HPLC

Analysis by reverse phase was performed in apparatus from Waters Ass. using the following modules: WISP 710A sample applicator, two pumps model 6000A, spectrophotometer model 440 using a 280 nm filter, the Data Module and the System Controller model 720.

Columns were thermostated at 30°C, except for one instance where HI and DAI were separated at 40°C.

Three brands of columns have been used. Initially 4 × 300 mm Water μBondpak C_{18} columns, 10 μm particle size, were used. This column, with virtually no free silanol groups, yields broad but symmetrical peaks. A 4 × 200 mm Nucleosil C_{18} 5–100 column, 5 μm particle size, has been used for most analyses because, despite incomplete coverage of silanol groups, sharp although not symmetrical peaks were obtained. Usually more than 2000 runs were achieved on a column. Eluents were generated by pump mixing of an aqueous solution of 0.4 M $(NH_4)_2SO_4$, pH adjusted to 3.5 with H_2SO_4 (B), with water/acetonitrile 1/1 parts per volume (A). Flow rate was usually 1 ml/min. For isocratic elution 51% A and 49% B permitted separation of DOI, DOI-Thr-OMe, PI and HI-OMe in 20–30 minutes. When the more hydrophobic human insulin esters HI-OBu^t and HI(Bu^t)-OBu^t were to be eluted a gradient up to 76 parts of A (38 parts CH_3CN) was generated during 25 minutes, using the formula (i) (Waters no. 7):

$$\text{(i)} \qquad \%A_t = \%A_0 + (\%A_w - \%A_0)\left[\frac{t - t_0}{t_w - t_0}\right]^2$$

where t, t_0 and t_w denote actual time, time for gradient start, and time for end of gradient, respectively, and A_t, A_0, and A_w denote the corresponding parts of A in the mixture at the indicated time. Using this concave gradient DAI (including PI) and HI-OMe are still separated, see Figures 5 and 6, and the hydrophobic HI(Bu^t)-OBu^t elutes towards the end of the gradient, followed by trypsin and its degradation products. Finally a 4.6 × 250 mm LiChrosorb RP-18 (5μ) column was used in one experiment in which HI and DAI were separated, Figure 8. For this separation isocratic elution was performed at 40°C with an eluent composed of an aqueous part of 0.1 M Na_2SO_4, 0.04 M H_3PO_4 titrated to pH 2.3 with ethanolamine and to which acetonitrile was added to about 30% (v/v).

Setting the integration parameters of the Data module to 25 s for the peak width and to 25 μV/s for the noise reduction, integration was achieved of peaks amounting to far less than 1% of the total (<2 μg) in the gradient system. Using isocratic elution, peaks of less than 1% and emerging after 15 min were too flat to be picked up using the above settings.

The samples of acetone or NaCl precipitated insulin compounds, usually 1.25 mg, were dissolved in 250 μl 1 M acetic acid, filtered through a 4 mm Millipore AP 25 filter, punched out and placed in the Luer fitting of a 0.45 × 10 mm hypodermic needle, using a 1 ml B-D polypropylene syringe to press the solution through the filter, and the plastic needle shield to hold the filtrate for insertion into the glass bottles of the carousel of the WISP

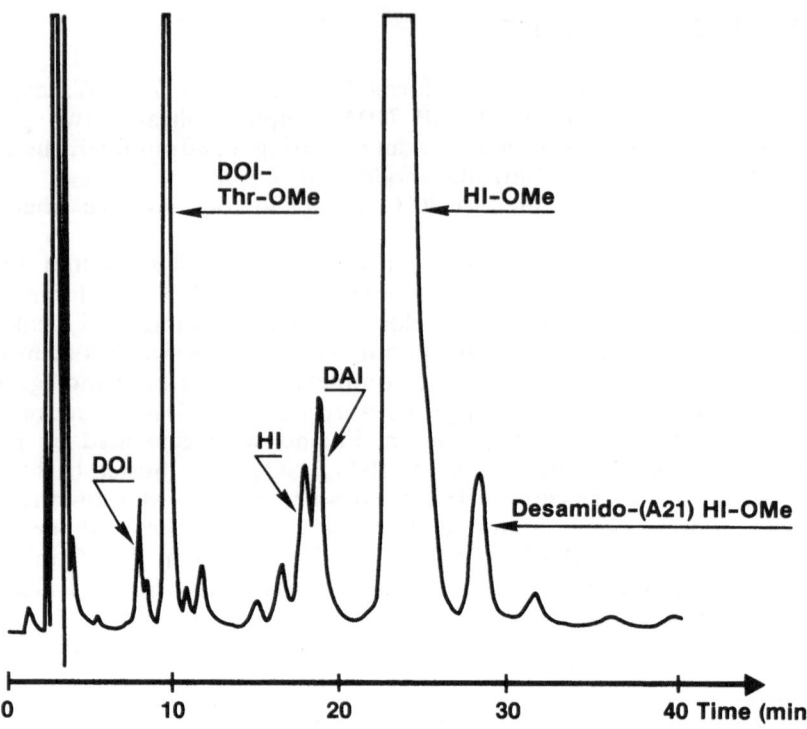

Figure 8 HPLC diagram of proteins from reaction mixture in which the equilibrium DAI + Thr-OMe ⇌ HI-OMe has been established (144 h). The HPLC system (LiChrosorb C_{18} column) provides for a separation of HI and DAI, the HI being formed by non-enzymatic hydrolysis of HI-OMe. Isocratic elution

automatic sample applicator. 50 μl, corresponding to 200 μg of insulin compounds, was injected.

Using the absorbance at 280 nm implies that it is mainly the four tyrosine residues of insulin that contribute to the signal. Hence the molar extinctions of porcine insulin and human insulin esters were taken to be identical. DOI and DOI-Thr-OR compounds have lost tyrosine B26. Consequently, integrated areas of these compounds were corrected by a factor of 1.33. This correction was not possible when separation was incomplete, e.g. in mixtures of DAI and DOI-Thr-OBu^t, and in mixtures of SCI and DOI-Thr-OMe.

The trypsin contained in the precipitated and redissolved samples is kept inactive in the 1 M acetic acid. A progressing deamidation of Asn^{A21} takes place in 1 M acetic acid in the WISP module, where the temperature exceeds 30°C. The desamido compounds elute immediately after the corresponding parent compounds. Another set of satellite peaks occurs if the organic solvents have contained trace amounts of aldehydes which have modified the N-terminal amino groups. In the calculation of yields such small and often unknown derivatives have been ignored. Yields were calculated by normalizing the integrated areas under the peaks, 'amounts', of the known compounds to 100%. Peaks of B-chain peptides B(23–30) and B(23–29)-Thr-OMe were excluded from the calculation, as the losses were compensated for by correcting DOI and DOI-Thr-OMe by a factor 1.33. In this way yields and losses after precipitation with NaCl, where the heptapeptide B(23–29) and the octapeptide B(23–29)-Thr-OMe are lost in the supernatant, can still be estimated.

A number of compounds coelute in HPLC. Porcine insulin and DAI coelute in the systems used here. Human insulin also coelutes with PI and DAI except when using the LiChrosorb column on which HI elutes slightly earlier than DAI, Figure 8. DOI-Thr-OBu^t elutes in a position just before DAI, and the peaks are resolved only when both are small, Figure 9. Early in the chromatograms, the order of elution is: DOI < SCI-AAK < SCI < DOI-Thr-OMe. Figure 10 shows an isocratic elution of a reaction mixture containing DOI and DOI-Thr-OMe, which has been spiked with SCI that elutes in between. The human insulin esters HI-OEt and HI-OMse elute just after HI-OMe, the order of elution being:

$$HI\text{-}OMe < HI\text{-}OMse < HI\text{-}OEt$$

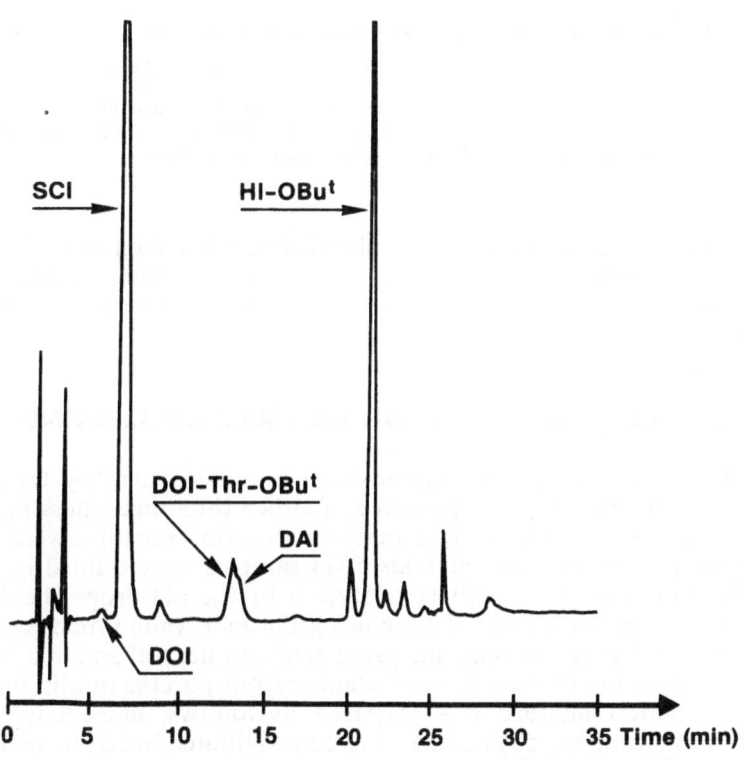

Figure 9 HPLC diagram of proteins in a reaction mixture from a conversion of SCI to HI-OBu^t. Note the overlapping peaks of DOI-Thr-OBu^t and DAI. Gradient elution

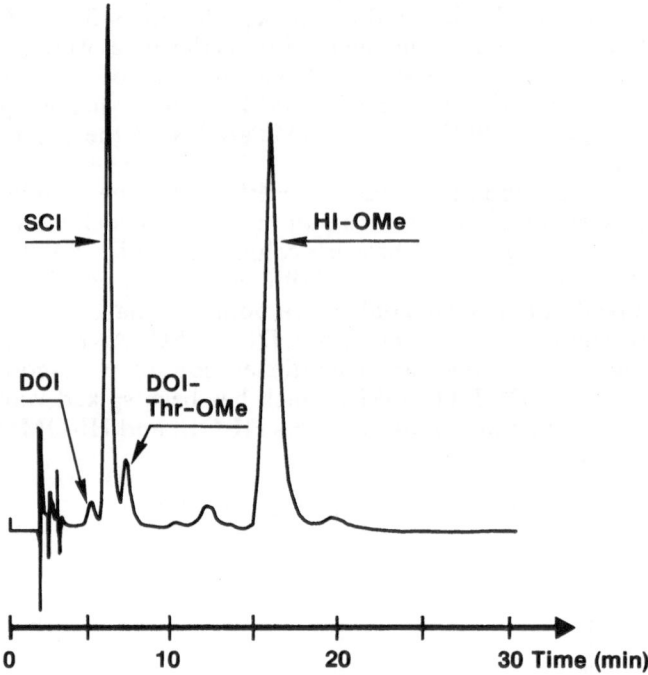

Figure 10 HPLC diagram of proteins in a reaction mixture from a conversion of porcine insulin to HI-OMe. The sample has been spiked with SCI to demonstrate the relative positions of SCI and the by-products DOI and DOI-Thr-OMe. Isocratic elution

Late in the chromatograms the hydrophobic human insulin esters HI(Bu^t)-OBu^t and HI-OTmb emerge, almost at the end of the gradient which lasts 25 min plus 3 min to account for the void volume, Figures 11 and 12, respectively.

9.   AMINO ACID ANALYSIS FOR RELEASE OF ALANINE

The kinetics of the release of alanine from porcine insulin by trypsin in organic–aqueous media in the presence of either threonine esters or other amines was assessed by amino acid analyses. Reaction mixtures were set up as described in section 1. At intervals 50 µl samples were diluted in 2.5 ml 0.026 N HCl to quench the activity of trypsin by the pH drop. The diluted samples were analysed for free alanine using the Jeol Amino Acid Analyzer, using a shortened program only analysing acid and neutral amino acids. An internal standard for 100% release of alanine from porcine insulin for each particular reaction mixture was prepared as follows: immediately after completion of the mixing 50 µl of the mixture was diluted in 1.25 ml of 60 mM Tris/5 mM calcium acetate in water and left at room temperature for 24 hours. Then 1.25 ml of 0.112 N HCl was added to establish the appropriate

36

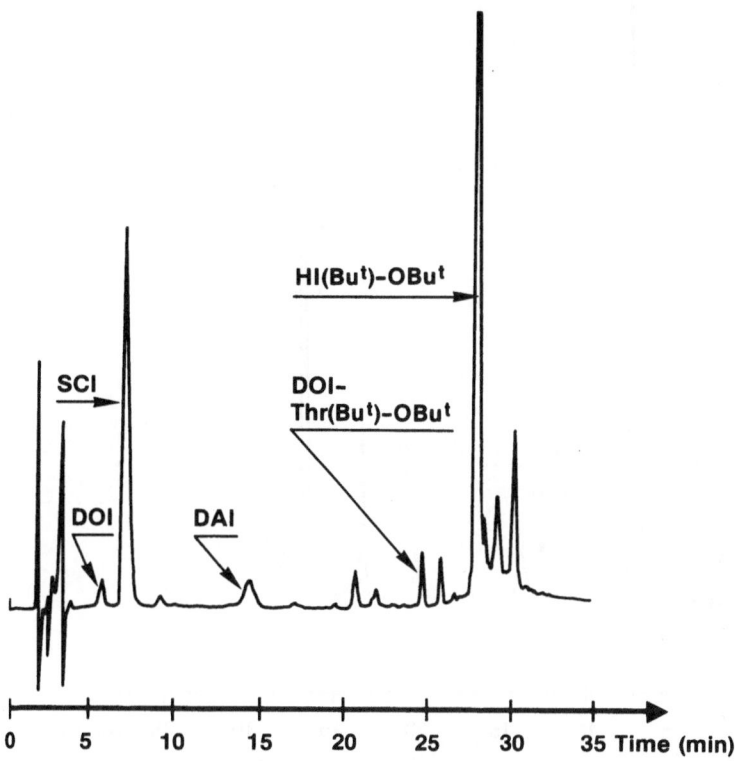

Figure 11 HPLC diagram of proteins in a reaction mixture from a conversion of SCI to HI(Buᵗ)-OBuᵗ. The by-products DOI and DOI-Thr(Buᵗ)-OBuᵗ are well separated from the DAI in equilibrium with HI(Buᵗ)-OBuᵗ. Gradient elution

pH for amino acid analysis. The resulting concentration of alanine released from porcine insulin in the '100% standard' with 8 mM porcine insulin in the reaction mixture is $= 8/51$ mM $= 157$ nmole/ml. Such values were found when the '100% standards' were compared to external alanine standards. The released alanine in the samples from the kinetic experiments is expressed as a percentage of the '100% standard'.

10. ANALYSIS FOR TRYPSIN ACTIVITY IN REACTION MIXTURES

The stability of trypsin as a function of acid/base ratio, percentage water and temperature in the organic–aqueous reaction mixtures was analysed by its amidase activity. Immediately after mixing as described in section 1, a 20 μl zero sample was diluted in 20 ml 0.2 M Tris, 0.01 M calcium chloride buffer, adjusted to pH 7.8 with HCl. After appropriate intervals and up to 48 h, 20 μl samples were withdrawn from the reaction mixtures and diluted in 20 ml of the Tris/CaCl$_2$ buffer. The amidase activity in the diluted samples

37

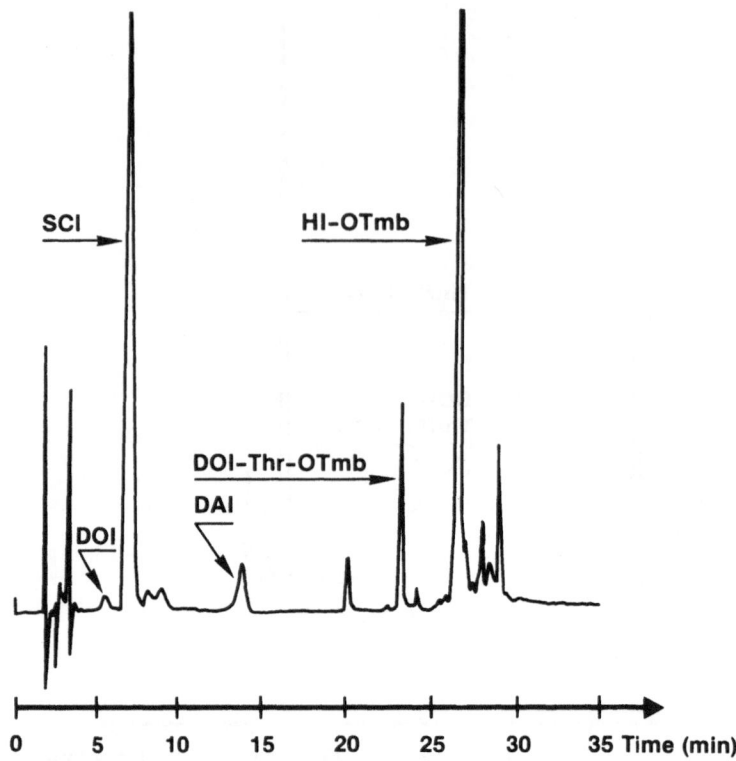

Figure 12 HPLC diagram of proteins in a reaction mixture from a conversion of SCI to HI-OTmb, showing the positions of by-products DOI and DOI-Thr-OTmb, and DAI in equilibrium with HI-OTmb. Gradient elution

was assessed immediately after dilution by mixing 2 ml with 1 ml Bz-D,L-Arg-*p*-nitroanilide solution (1 mg BAPA/ml of water, dissolved by heating) and following the increase in extinction at 405 nm for 10–15 min. The reference cell contained a mixture of 2 ml Tris/CaCl$_2$ buffer and 1 ml BAPA solution. Solutions were thermostated at 25°C. The trypsin activity expressed as increase in absorbance units cm^{-1} min^{-1} was calculated from the measurements by the method of the least squares. In the dilutions at time zero where the estimated trypsin concentrations were $0.2 \times 1/1001 \times 2/3$ mM $= 0.133\,\mu$M, the trypsin activity (A_0) was found to be 0.062 ± 0.004 SEM absorbance units cm^{-1} min^{-1}. The method as applied here is a modification from Erlanger *et al.*[105], as developed in the Enzyme Chemistry Laboratories, Novo.

The autolysis of trypsin in aqueous solutions has been shown by Lazdunski and Delaage[106] to follow 2nd order kinetics. Hence the rate constants for trypsin autolysis in the organic–aqueous media were calculated as second-order rate constants from (ii):

(ii)
$$k_a = \frac{(A_0 - A_t)}{T_0 \times t \times A_t} = \frac{(A_0 - A_t)}{0.2 \times t \times A_t}\,\text{mM}^{-1}\,\text{h}^{-1}$$

where k_a is the second-order rate constant, t the time, and A_0 and A_t the activity at time zero and t, respectively, and T_0 initial trypsin concentration $= 0.2\,\text{mM}$.

The initial rate of autolysis V_0 is (iii):

(iii) $$V_0 = k_a T_0^2 = 0.04 \times k_a\,\text{mM}\,\text{h}^{-1} = 20 \times k_a\,\%\,\text{h}^{-1}$$

Although the trypsin activity decayed in a hyperbolic fashion typical of 2nd order reactions, the k_a values at various times did not fit equation (ii) satisfactorily well to propose second order kinetics for the autolysis of trypsin in organic–aqueous media. Wu et al.[107] reported a perfect second-order denaturation of α-trypsin at neutral pH in aqueous solution and a more complex reaction for the autolysis of β-trypsin possibly involving a conformational change, cleavage to α-trypsin and, finally, second-order cannibalistic autolysis. A similar complexity in organic–aqueous media is therefore not surprising. The 'second-order' k_a values have been estimated from readings where $0.25\,A_0 < A_t < 0.75\,A_0$. They shall only serve as indicators when comparing the stability of trypsin at various conditions in such media.

3
The specificity

1. A MODEL FOR TWO SITES OF CLEAVAGE

The specificity becomes a topic in the tryptic transpeptidation of insulins as both Arg^{B22} and Lys^{B29} are cleavage sites. Reaction at arginine leads irreversibly to desoctapeptide insulin (DOI) and, in the presence of Thr-OR, to DOI-Thr^{B23}-OR, and such products represent losses. Reaction at lysine leads to des(Ala^{B30}) insulin and, in the presence of Thr-OR, to the corresponding human insulin ester. The product, HI-OR, is still substrate for the side reaction at Arg^{B22} and the yield of the product will reach a maximum dependent only upon the ratio between the two rate constants, which we will denote the specificity, q.

Let A be the starting material, B the product and C the by-product:

(i) $$A \xrightarrow{k_B} B$$

(ii) $$A \xrightarrow{k_C} C$$

(iii) $$B \xrightarrow{k_C} C$$

Provided the enzyme is stable under the reaction conditions, the rate equations become:

(iv) $$\frac{dA}{dt} = -A(k_B + k_C)$$

(v) $$\frac{dB}{dt} = k_B A - k_C B$$

(vi) $$\frac{dC}{dt} = k_C(A + B)$$

The rate constant for formation of C, k_C, is assumed to be independent of whether the substrate for formation of C is A or B. This assumption is presumably valid in the case of insulin, the cleavage site B22–B23 being separated by seven residues from B29–B30. Hence cleavage at B(22–23) is considered to be independent of the presence of residue B30.

40

The solutions of the rate equations are:

(vii)
$$A = A_0 e^{-(k_B + k_C)t}$$

(viii)
$$B = A_0 e^{-k_C t}(1 - e^{-k_B t})$$

(ix)
$$C = A_0(1 - e^{-k_C t})$$

The yield of B has its maximum at $t = t_{max}$

(x)
$$t_{max} = \frac{\ln[(k_B + k_C)/k_C]}{k_B}$$

The maximum yield of $B = B_{max}$ becomes:

(xi)
$$B_{max} = A_0 e^{-(k_C/k_B)\ln(1 + k_B/k_C)}(1 - e^{-\ln(1 + k_B/k_C)})$$

Inserting the specificity $q = k_B/k_C$ in (xi) gives:

(xii)
$$B_{max} = A_0(1 + q)^{-q^{-1}}(1 - 1/(1 + q)) = A_0 q/[(1 + q)^{1 + q^{-1}}]$$

In this case, where the product B enters an equilibrium between human insulin ester and des-(B30) insulin, the yield B represents the sum of the two species in equilibrium.

The maximum attainable yield (B_{max}) as a function of q is given in Table 4, and depicted in Figure 13. Note that a specificity of 100 is required to attain a yield of 95%, and with a specificity of 1 the maximum yield is 25%. A major task of the experimental work was to find conditions where the specificity q is satisfactorily high.

The ratio between starting material A and by-product C at the time when the product B reaches its maximum is:

(xiii)
$$A/C(t_{max}) = \frac{1}{(1 + q)[(1 + q)^{q^{-1}} - 1]}$$

A/C (t_{max}) as a function of q is shown in Table 4 and depicted in Figure 13. Note how insensitive A/C (t_{max}) is to variations in q in the interesting area with yields higher than 90%, corresponding to q larger than about 50. If a synthesis with such a q value is monitored and stopped when A/C is about 0.2, the yield B is very near B_{max}.

The specificity q using a single sample of a reaction mixture containing the mole fractions A, B and C of substrate, product and by-product, respectively, is calculated according to (xiv):

(xiv)
$$q = \frac{k_B}{k_C} = \frac{\ln\left[\dfrac{A}{A + B}\right]}{\ln(A + B)} = \frac{\ln\left[\dfrac{A}{1 - C}\right]}{\ln(A + B)}$$

using $A + B + C = 1$. If the rate constants k_B and k_C are determined from separate samples taken at times t' and t'', respectively, the calculation of q

Yield, mole fraction

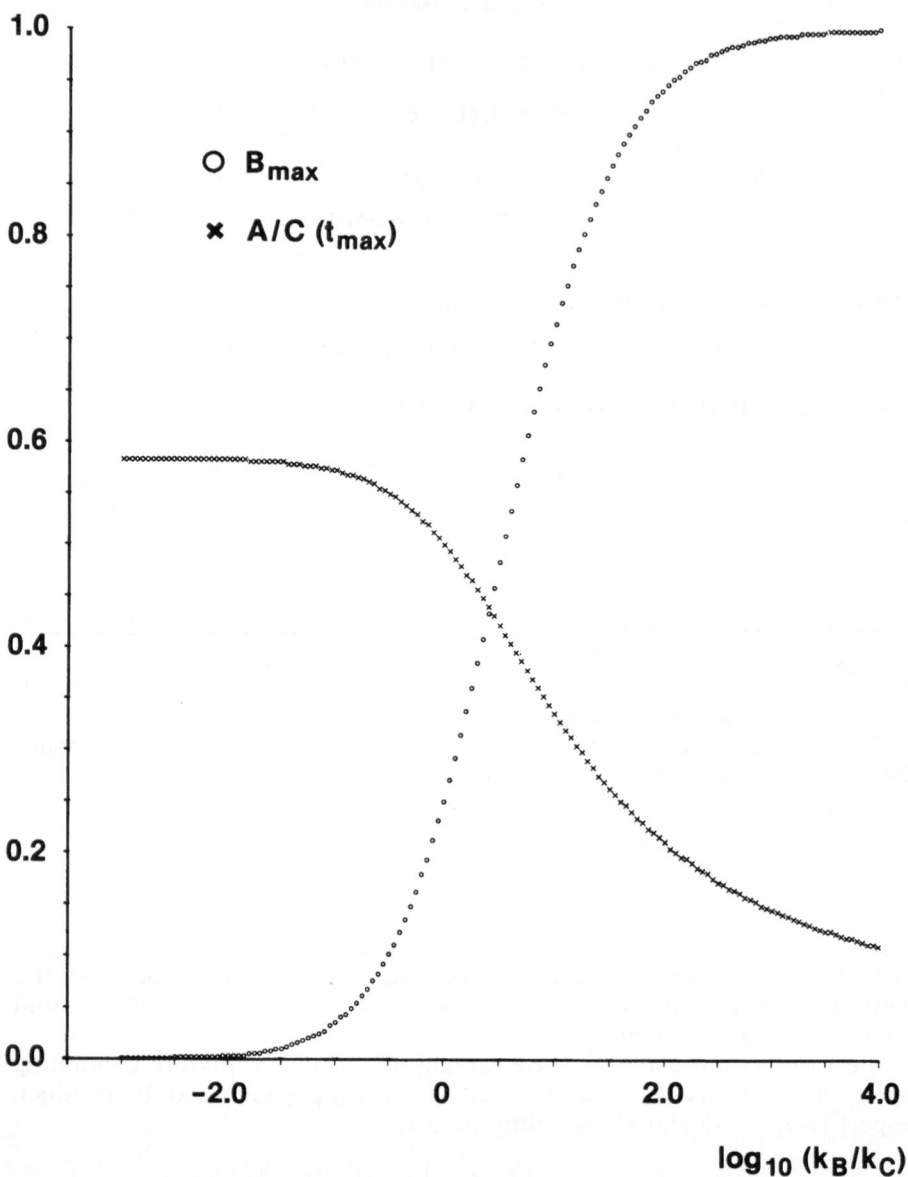

Figure 13 Plot of the maximum yield B_{max} (circles) and the ratio between starting material A and by-product C at the time t_{max} where yields are at maximum (crosses) as a function of the specificity $q = k_B/k_C$, viz. the ratio between two rate constants

is performed according to (xv):

(xv)
$$q = \frac{k_B}{k_C} = \frac{t'' \ln\left[\dfrac{A_{t''}}{1 - C_{t'}}\right]}{t' \ln(A_{t''} + B_{t''})}$$

Formula (xv) finds application when the rate constants differ markedly, viz. when $k_B \gg k_C$.

4
Transpeptidation of porcine insulin to human insulin esters

1. INTRODUCTION

The yield in the transpeptidation reaction depends on four physicochemically controlled variables, the displacement of the equilibria in equation (i), the formation of by-products, the rate of reactions and the stability of the enzyme.

$$\text{Porcine insulin} \xrightarrow{-\text{Ala}} \text{DAI-trypsin} \underset{\pm \text{Thr-OR}}{\rightleftharpoons} \text{HI-OR}$$

(i)
$$\underset{\pm \text{H}_2\text{O}\,\uparrow\downarrow}{}$$
$$\text{DAI}$$

The variables depend, in turn, on a variety of factors like temperature, time, type of solvent, content of water, acid/base ratio, type of threonine ester and counter ions. The interplay by which all these factors influence the variables to bring about the yield becomes intricate. Separation of the variables is not always possible, for instance, where a by-product is not separated from the starting material in the analysis (by-product formation or enzyme inactivation) or when a by-product is not separated from DAI (by-product formation or unfavourable equilibrium). The ratio between the rates of the forward reaction (i) and trypsin inactivation is of decisive importance to the yields. By-products form either due to lack of specificity in the enzymatic reaction, or because the product is chemically unstable, e.g. human insulin methyl ester is being hydrolysed to human insulin which, in turn, is transpeptidized back to human insulin methyl ester as long as the trypsin is still active, (ii):

(ii)
$$\text{Porcine insulin} \xrightarrow[+\text{Thr-OMe}]{-\text{Ala}} \text{HI-OMe} \xrightarrow[+\text{H}_2\text{O}]{-\text{CH}_3\text{OH}} \text{HI}$$

$$\xrightarrow[+\text{Thr-OMe}]{-\text{Thr}} \text{HI-OMe}$$

Human insulin formed in the transpeptidation reaction is a by-product, as it cannot be separated from either porcine insulin or DAI by the preparative means available today. Due to the intricacy and interplay of variables that determine yields, most investigators have reported yields of human insulin esters only and abstained from comments as to the causes.

2. STABILITY OF TRYPSIN IN ORGANIC–AQUEOUS MEDIA

Harris[104] described the inactivation of trypsin in 8 M urea solutions as a reversible unfolding. At intermediate urea concentrations irreversible inactivation progresses because, in an equilibrium between active trypsin and inactive, unfolded molecules, the latter become substrate for the active trypsin molecules. A similar mechanism was expected to be active when using other organic solvents than urea. Inouye et al.[108] demonstrated that addition of organic solvents, such as DMF and DMSO, had a stabilizing effect on trypsin in the absence of Ca^{2+} up to about 30–50% organic solvent. It was argued that the diminution of catalytic efficiency caused by addition of organic solvents also prevents the autocatalytic digestion which occurs in the absence of Ca^{2+}. At higher concentrations the stability of trypsin decreases with increasing concentration of organic solvent. In the presence of 10 mM Ca^{2+} the lowest stability was found at the highest concentrations of organic solvents, most pronounced in DMF/BD (1/1) and in BD. Of the various organic solvents, BD and mixtures thereof with DMF and DMSO result in the highest rate of trypsin inactivation in the presence of Ca^{2+}. In all cases Ca^{2+} ions had a stabilizing influence on trypsin. The apparent discrepancy between the two studies may be due to the difference in temperatures, concentration of calcium or type of solvent. The studies in urea were conducted at 20°C, and the studies in various organic solvents at 30°C.

In the present investigation the stability of trypsin in aqueous DMAC was studied in a complete $3 \times 3 \times 3$ factorial experiment, the factors being temperature, % water and acid/base ratio (Table 5). The data have been fitted to the second-order model for trypsin autolysis by Lazdunski and Delaage[106] but the fit suggested that the model only describes the autolysis in qualitative terms. Nevertheless, the second-order rate constant of autolysis, k_a, was preferred as the way to represent the stability data most comprehensibly (Table 5). The first-order denaturation of trypsin in urea described by Delaage and Lazdunski[109] complied less well with these data in DMAC than the second-order model. Increasing the temperature greatly decreases stability, and a large gain in stability is obtained by lowering the temperature from 25°C to 12°C. The increase in stability gained by a decrease in temperature abundantly compensates for the decrease in reaction rates of trypsin catalysed couplings and transpeptidations. At 12 and 25°C the stability increases as the water content increases from 20% to 30%, in accordance with the data of Inouye et al.[108]. However, at 38°C the stability decreases as the water content increases, which parallels the urea induced autolysis[104]. Lowering the pH in aqueous solutions is known to stabilize trypsin[106]. The stabilizing effect of acid is also effective in DMAC solutions (Table 5). A marked decrease in k_a is found between the acetic acid/acetate 0/1 (M/M) buffer and the more acidic 1.5/1 (M/M) buffer, about a factor 4 at 12°C. A smaller difference is seen between the H^+-Thr-OMe/Thr-OMe 0.5/0.5 (M/M) buffer and the HOAc/OAc⁻ 0/1 (M/M) buffer, about a factor 2 at 12°C.

A k_a of $0.055\,h^{-1}\,mM^{-1}$ is found at the set of conditions that was selected for the kinetic studies, viz. 20.7% water, 12°C, HOAc/OAc⁻ 1.5/1.0 (M/M), 0.2 mM trypsin and 3 mM Ca^{2+}. The initial autolysis of trypsin is estimated to be $k_a \times T^2 = 0.0022\,mM/h$, corresponding to $1.1\%\,h^{-1}$.

Indirectly the instability of trypsin can be evaluated by inadequate establishment of equilibrium and by a stop in by-product formation. The stabilizing effect of calcium ions on trypsin activity in organic–aqueous medium was seen in coupling and transpeptidation reactions that slowed down and stopped early in the absence of Ca^{2+}. Furthermore, the formation of the by-products DOI and DOI-Thr[B23]-OR often continued in the presence of Ca^{2+}, whereas this was not the case in the absence of Ca^{2+}, confirming the stabilizing effect of Ca^{2+} on trypsin. Results from multifactor experiments where Ca^{2+} was a factor are shown in Tables 6–11. The right timing of trypsin inactivation at 37°C due to the absence of Ca^{2+} results in the highest yield (83%) in one experiment (Table 6). At 25°C the stabilizing effect of Ca^{2+} cannot be demonstrated in this medium, rich in BD, a solvent which was claimed to stabilize trypsin[108]. Note also the drop in yield at 37°C from 24 to 96 h, a result of hydrolysis of HI-OMe to HI. At 25°C the yields decrease from 24 to 96 h as a consequence of the continued action of trypsin forming DOI and DOI-Thr-OMe, indicating that the specificity of trypsin in the system is low.

In an ethanol medium containing 2 M acetic acid trypsin is inactivated in less than 30 min at 25°C in the absence of Ca^{2+}, before the coupling of DAI and Thr-OMe has reached equilibrium with HI-OMe (Table 7). The inactivation in the absence of calcium is enhanced in 11.8% water as compared to 16.6% water.

Table 8 shows a $2 \times 3 \times 3$ factorial coupling experiment in which three solvents, three temperatures and the presence and absence of Ca^{2+} are the factors. The effect of Ca^{2+} stabilization is most pronounced at higher temperatures. With a fixed content of water (20.9%) the instability in the absence of Ca^{2+} increases through the series:

$$DMAC < BD < ethanol$$

The declining yields at 37°C as a function of time are caused by hydrolysis of HI-OMe to HI.

The stabilization of trypsin is more critical for transpeptidation than for coupling, as transpeptidation reactions are slower than coupling reactions. The effect of Ca^{2+} appears most pronounced at low concentrations of trypsin (Table 9). Again, the inactivation of trypsin in the absence of Ca^{2+} is also in DMAC most pronounced at the low level of water concentration.

Neither addition of zinc ions, TPCK treatment of trypsin nor the purity of porcine insulin appeared to influence the stability of trypsin (Table 10). Stabilization by Ca^{2+} in this highly aqueous medium has an adverse effect on the yields as by-product formation becomes prevalent.

The inactivation of trypsin as a function of water concentration and of temperature in four aprotic solvents can be inferred from the yields in Table 11. The more rapid inactivation at higher temperature and at lower concentrations of water was shown already in Tables 5, 7, 8 and 9. The data in the presence of Ca^{2+} at 13.4% water in Table 11 suggest a ranking of the solvents according to power to inactivate trypsin:

$$DMSO > NMP > DMF > DMAC$$

From Table 8 the ranking inferred at 20.9% water in the absence of Ca^{2+} was:

$$Ethanol > BD > DMAC$$

Unique among the solvents is 1,4-butanediol in that it permits trypsin catalysed reaction at water concentrations down to about 3%, see Rose and Offord[75] and Table 6.

To sum up: in the range of water concentrations of special interest for trypsin catalysed reactions (around 20%) trypsin is stabilized by:

(a) addition of Ca^{2+} ions
(b) low temperature
(c) increased concentration of water
(d) increased acidity
(e) use of DMAC as the organic solvent rather than alcohols.

3. FACTORS INFLUENCING THE SPECIFICITY OF TRYPSIN

Markussen[65] stated that a low content of water and a high content of acid in the transpeptidation reaction mixture decreased the by-product formation. More specifically, two significant factors for the specificity, as defined in Chapter 3, are water concentration and acidity. In addition lowering the temperature increases specificity, and the type of organic solvent is also an important factor. Factorial experiments from which the influence of the parameters on the trypsin specificity q can be deduced are compiled in Tables 12–31. In many cases reactions were approaching equilibrium before the first sampling, and then the estimate of q derived from the data represents a minimum value.

The interplay of the water concentration and the acidity factor on the yield in one preferred solvent, DMAC, is shown in Tables 12–16. At the higher concentrations of water and at low acidity the yields drop due to lack of specificity, i.e. transpeptidation or hydrolysis at Arg^{B22}. On the other hand, at the lower concentration of water and at high acidity reactions come to a stop due to trypsin inactivation. Tables 12, 13 and 14 show data from experiments at 37°C. As the trypsin is usually inactivated before the equilibrium has been established at 37°C these data are suitable to demonstrate the interplay. At about 30% water the inactivation of trypsin precedes the transpeptidation resulting in low yields. The highest value of q found at 37°C is 66 (Table 14) using 27.9% H_2O in acetic acid/acetate 0.25/1 (M/M). A maximum yield of 92% HI-OMe can be estimated from Figure 13, provided that trypsin could be preserved in an active form and that the equilibrium between DAI and HI-OMe (i) is virtually completely displaced towards HI-OMe.

Since both lower water concentrations and higher acidity cause the specificity q to increase and, on the other hand, such changes make trypsin unstable, the means to overcome the dilemma was to lower the temperature. In spite of this obvious possibility, most workers in the field[41,56,60,63,73,75] conducted reactions at room temperature or at 37°C. Tables 15 and 16 show yields of HI-OMe (α) and specificities (q) obtained at 12°C and 18°C. At 12°C trypsin is stabilized to the extent that reactions can be carried out down to about 17% H_2O in DMAC, using an acetic acid/acetate 1.5/1 (M/M) buffer. Values of q in the order of 200–400 can be estimated, corresponding to yields up to 98% (Figure 13), the provision being the complete displacement of the equilibrium (i) towards synthesis.

The yields at 12°C in Tables 15 and 16 have been interpolated in order to construct the 90% iso-yield contour-line for transpeptidation (Figure 14). The corresponding graph for coupling reactions covers a larger area and confines that of transpeptidation in all directions, as coupling reactions proceed faster than transpeptidations. In the calculation of q use has been made of the early observations in the calculation of $k(Lys^{B29})$ and late observations in the calculation of $k(Arg^{B22})$ in those cases where by-product formation is slow. The precision of the estimated q values is not high, but ample to describe the pronounced importance of the water concentration and acidity of the medium. In the use of q the assumption is made that it remains constant as long as the trypsin is active. Partly degraded but still active forms of trypsin (α-trypsin, γ-trypsin) could have a changed specificity. No consistent indication of such a change can be deduced from the data, but in solvents composed of organic solids dissolved in water the specificity appears to decrease with time (Tables 29 and 30).

Indirectly, an increase in specificity is gained by lowering the temperature because the increase in stability of trypsin permits a decrease in water concentration and an increase in acidity. But does the temperature itself influence the specificity? Table 17 shows the data from a transpeptidation experiment in water concentrations ranging from 23.6 to 27.8% at 23, 31 and 37°C. The q values increase with decreasing temperature, but the correlation appears insignificant when related to the precision of the q values. Likewise, in Table 18, data from transpeptidations in water concentrations ranging from 13.5 to 29.4% at 7 and 12°C fail to disclose any such correlation. However, by increasing the water concentration to 35% (Table 19) and 44.8% (Table 20) and expanding the temperature range to the interval -18 to 60°C, a striking effect of the temperature on the specificity is demonstrated. Transpeptidations highly specific at Lys^{B29} can be conducted at -10 and -18°C in media that at higher temperatures render but little protection against reaction at Arg^{B22}. No search was made to find any lower temperature limit for tryptic action, but it appears as if the catalysis may proceed until the mixture solidifies.

The ability of three other threonine esters, Thr-OEt, Thr-O(CH$_2$)$_2$SO$_2$CH$_3$ and Thr(Bu^t)-OBu^t, to induce specificity in the transpeptidation reaction was

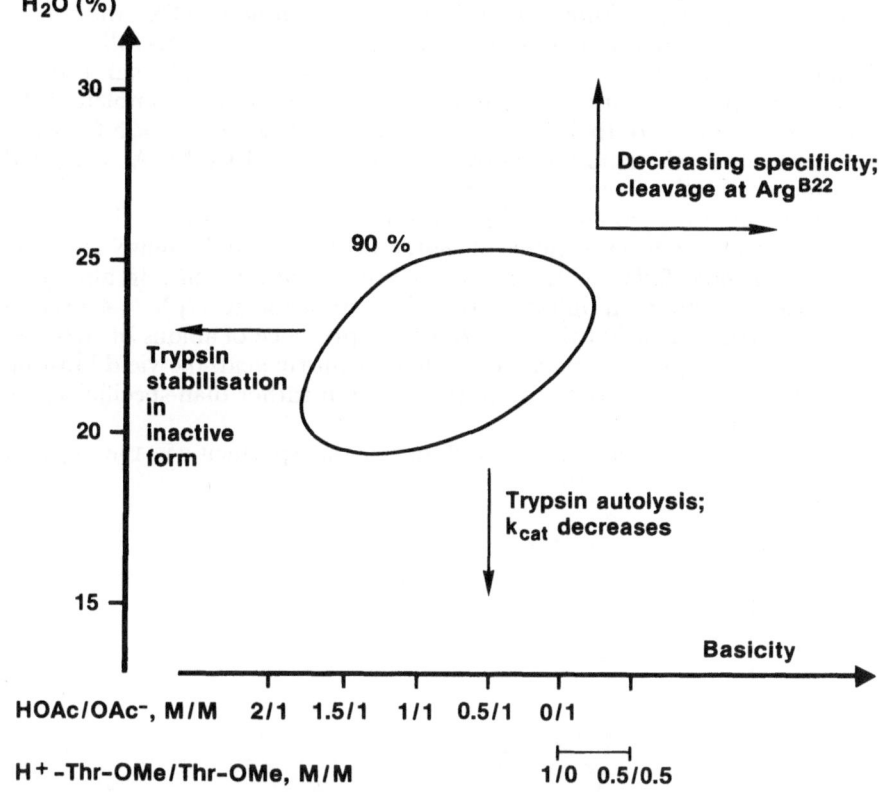

Figure 14 The 90% iso-yield curve for transpeptidation of porcine insulin to human insulin methyl ester as a function of basicity (x-axis) and water content (y-axis) of the reaction medium. The arrows show why yields decrease by a change in the indicated direction. The iso-yield curve is found at 12°C, using DMAC as the organic solvent and 1 M Thr-OMe. Data refer to Tables 15 and 16

tested under various concentrations of water and in various acetic acid/acetate buffers (Table 21). Due to low solubility Thr-O(CH$_2$)$_2$SO$_2$CH$_3$ was assayed at concentrations of 0.33 M and below. With none of these esters were specificities achieved comparable to those obtained with Thr-OMe (Tables 15 and 16), but the conditions of assaying are not exactly identical. As the esters in the concentrations used here contribute substantially to the volume of the mixture (5–20%, v/v) it is conceivable that they influence the specificity either by a direct solvent effect or indirectly by the volume of DMAC that they replace.

In the crystallographic hexameric unit of 2-zinc insulin crystals, two Zn^{2+} each coordinate three imidazole groups from 3 His^{B10} residues belonging to three different insulin dimeric subunits, *vide* Baker *et al.*[110]. In aqueous solutions in the presence of zinc the hexameric unit is the preferred conformation in the neutral pH range[111]. Any influence of zinc should be abolished in mixtures of water and organic solvents, where dissociation to

49

the insulin monomer is known to occur. One example is 60% ethanol, as used in the chromatographic purification of insulin by Schlichtkrull et al.[93], and another example is 26% acetonitrile as used in analytical HPLC. Nonetheless, an investigation of insulin reactivity would be incomplete if the zinc factor was omitted. In Table 22 the result is shown of a 2×5 factorial experiment where the zinc concentrations were 0 and 6 mM. As expected zinc influences neither reaction progress nor the specificity.

Propionic acid/propionate buffers were compared to acetic acid/acetate buffers at various concentrations of water (Table 23 and Figure 15). The present experiment failed to reveal any possible real difference in ability to induce specificity between buffers of the stronger acetic acid (pK = 4.75) and the weaker propionic acid (pK = 4.87). In the presence of anions of stronger acids (formic acid, phosphoric acid and hydrochloric acid) the yield limiting causes are reaction rates and trypsin inactivation rather than specificity, see section 6 of this chapter.

The fourth major factor which influences the specificity is the type of

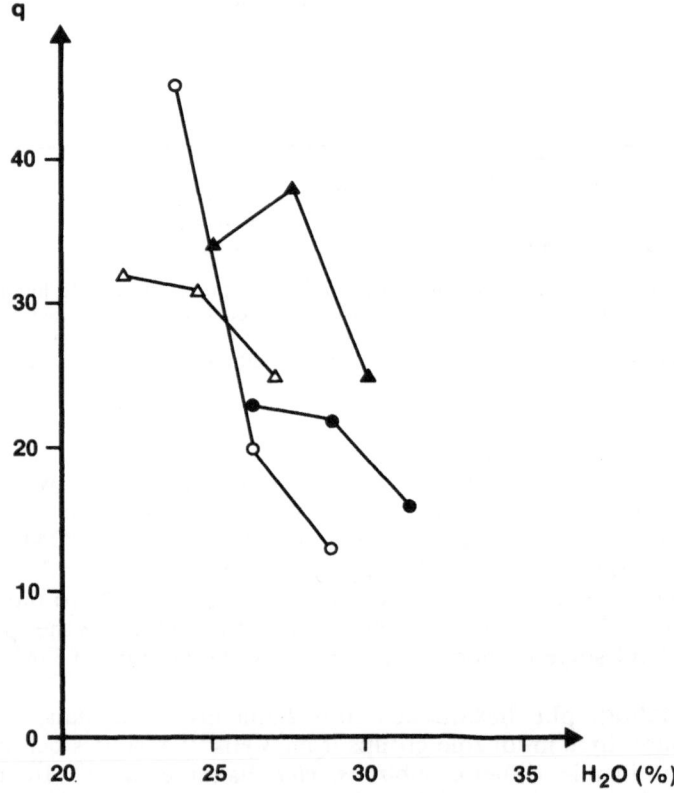

Figure 15 Plot of the specificity q ($= k_B/k_C$) as a function of water concentration, comparing propionic acid (open symbols) with acetic acid (closed symbols). Acid/base: 0.5/1 (M/M) circles; 0.73/1 (M/M) triangles. Results refer to Table 23

solvent. Highest specificities were found in strongly polar, aprotic solvents such as DMF and DMAC. Table 24 shows the results of a $2 \times 3 \times 4$ factorial experiment (temperature, water concentration and type of solvent), the four solvents being DMAC, DMF, THF and acetone. Due to limited solubility of Thr-OMe in THF the concentration is only 0.75 M in this solvent. For the same concentration of water the ranking of ability to induce specificity appears to be:

$$DMAC > DMF > acetone$$

Since initial observations are missing the apparent differences in specificity could also reflect differences in reaction rates, as reactions run faster in DMF than in DMAC, see in particular results at $-22°C$. As will be shown in Chapter 5, reactions proceed similarly in DMF and DMAC if the water concentration in the latter is about 3% higher. Likewise, the apparent large influence of temperature on specificity in this experiment may be due to lack of early observations for use in the calculation of $k(Lys^{B29})$.

Reaction rates are high in methanol and ethanol, and even the analysis at 4 h does not permit evaluation of the specificity (Table 25). In ethylene glycol and in glycerol the reaction rates are moderate, and specificities could be assessed. Experiments in DMAC under otherwise close to identical conditions are found in Tables 16 and 18. It is evident that for similar concentrations of water and buffer compositions, DMAC provides a higher specificity than these two alcohols. On the other hand, transpeptidation proceeds in ethylene glycol down to 11% water and in BD down to 4.8% water (Table 26), in agreement with Rose et al.[75]. Nevertheless, even in 4.8% water in BD and using equivalent amounts of acetic acid and Thr(Bu^t)-OBu^t the specificity is not especially high (Table 26). Moreover unknown peaks were observed in the HPLC chromatograms using alcohols as the organic solvent, presumably due to the corresponding esters of DAI and DOI (see comments on Tables 25 and 26).

The excess of threonine ester may itself serve as the organic solvent, although for industrial purposes it appears to represent an expensive choice[66,72]. Table 27 shows the results of transpeptidation experiments at various concentrations of water, in various buffers and at different temperatures, using Thr(Bu^t)-OBu^t as solvent. The usual pattern, described already for the dependence of the specificity upon these three factors, is also valid for this solvent.

Finally, a variety of organic compounds were tested for their ability as solvents to bring about transpeptidation of porcine insulin to human insulin ester and to induce specificity. The solids were urea and acetamide alone, and additions of phenol, guanidinium hydrochloride, ethanol, DMAC and polyethylene glycol to solutions of acetamide in water. The results are compiled in Tables 28–31. In no case were satisfactory yields obtained, one obstacle being that even in close to saturated solutions of the compounds the water concentrations were still too high. In urea solutions the concentration of water could be reduced to about 50% (Table 28). The yields were poor, most likely due to trypsin inactivation since DOI and DOI-Thr-OMe formation was low. Acetamide proved to be the most promising of the solids tested

(Table 29). The water concentration could be decreased to about 30% in this solvent, and yields of 60% were recorded. The specificities are not up to those found in DMAC, which in part is due to a decrease in $k(Lys^{B29})$. In polyethylene glycol (Macrogol 4000) the water concentration was reduced to about 30% (Table 30). Even with a ratio of acetic acid to acetate of 2/1 (M/M) the specificity was low and, accordingly, the yields too. No attempt was made to examine whether the trypsin had been inactivated after 48 h or whether the equilibrium constant $K_e(IM)$ in acetamide and polyethylene glycol is, in fact, largely reduced compared to that in DMAC (*vide* Tables 29 and 30 and compare to Tables 15 and 16). It is, in particular, in these solvents composed of solids dissolved in water that the assumption of a constant value for the specificity during the reaction progress appears questionable.

In order to further decrease the concentration of water in acetamide solutions, phenol, guanidinium hydrochloride, ethanol, DMAC and poly-ethylene glycol were added to a solution of acetamide containing 31.4% of water (Table 31). Both addition of phenol and guanidinium hydrochloride inhibit synthesis efficiently, probably through trypsin inactivation. Addition of 10% of either ethanol or DMAC has little or no effect on the yields. Only addition of 20 and 30% polyethylene glycol to the acetamide solution rendering water concentrations of 25 and 22% has a beneficial effect upon the yields.

In summary, four factors important for the specificity of the transpeptid-ation reaction at Lys^{B29} have been elucidated:

(a) The concentration of water; the lower the concentration, the higher the specificity.

(b) The acidity of the medium; the more acidic, the higher the specificity.

(c) The temperature; the lower the temperature, the higher the specificity.

(d) The type of organic solvent used to decrease the concentration of water; the strongly polar, aprotic solvents providing a higher specificity than alcohols.

Is the effect induced by these factors on the specificity due to changes in the insulin molecule and/or to changes in the trypsin molecule? Wang and Carpenter[61] demonstrated that the ratio between the rates of trypsin hydrolysis of the Arg-Gly (B22-B23) and the Lys-Ala (B29-B30) bonds is increased in oxidized B-chain as compared to intact insulin, suggesting a steric hindrance in intact insulin. Similarly, the rate of transpeptidation of the Lys-Gly (B29-A1) bond of the single-chain des-(B30) insulin molecule is markedly reduced as compared to that of the Lys-Ala (B29-B30) bond of porcine insulin, *vide* Chapter 5, again pointing to insulin conformation playing an important role for the specificity. In 'The structure of 2 Zn pig insulin crystals at 1.5 Å resolution'[110] the following interactions for residue Arg^{B22} are described based on the X-ray crystallographic studies:

'The residue NH is in a $1 \rightarrow 4$ turn formed at the end of the B9–B19 helix, with similar geometry in both molecules; the peptide O is directed into solvent and H bonded to 3 waters. The sidechain lies on the surface and is disordered with two fairly well defined principal conformations related by 180° rotation about C_γ-C_δ. Both conformations make salt bridges: one to the A21 carboxylic acid, the other to A17Glu carboxylic acid. The second arrangement also brings N_ε into H-bonding interaction with B18 O perhaps cancelling the negative charge produced there by the helix dipole (Hol, *Nature* 1979). In molecule 2, there is a salt bridge to B30 O_ε related by the threefold screw axis. Some well defined complementary water molecules, displaced from H bond interactions by the disordered guanidinium group, have been identified (7 w1 and 64 w1). In spite of the disorder, the two residues obey the local twofold axis quite well.'

Although such fixed structures, found in the hexameric unit cell in the crystalline state, are disrupted by dissolution in organic–aqueous media where the monomer is the predominant species, it could be argued that the salt bridge formed by the guanidinium group of Arg^{B22} and the neighbouring carboxyl group of Glu^{B21} is strengthened by the organic solvents rendering an increase of the K_m value, viz. increased dissociation from trypsin. However, the effect of the less polar alcohols to induce specificity should then be larger than that of the highly polar amide solvents, contrary to the findings. Hence a more likely but less specific explanation of the findings could be that a gross conformational change is induced in insulin by the polar aprotic solvents rendering Arg-Gly (B22-B23) less susceptible to trypsin.

Changes may also be induced in the trypsin by addition of organic solvents. A common feature appears to be that the specificity is low in solvents donating hydrogen for hydrogen bonding like formamide, acetamide, alcohols and water, and high in solvents accepting hydrogen in the formation of hydrogen bonds like DMF and DMAC. In early experiments using formamide in 43% water and acetic acid/acetate buffers at 37°C, neither HI-OMe nor DOI formation was observed using disc electrophoresis (Figure 16), indicating trypsin inactivation in this solvent. A change in the hydrogen bonds of the active site of trypsin could thus be made accountable for both the specificity changes observed and the destabilization of trypsin.

4. THE THERMODYNAMIC EQUILIBRIUM

Experiments at conditions where the trypsin stability is high are useful for the estimation of the equilibrium constants of the reactions (iii) and (iv):

(iii) $\underset{1-\alpha}{DAI} + Thr\text{-}OR \rightleftharpoons \underset{\alpha}{HI\text{-}OR} + H_2O$

(iv) $\underset{\beta_1}{DOI} + Thr\text{-}OR \rightleftharpoons \underset{\beta_2}{DOI\text{-}Thr\text{-}OR} + H_2O$

The apparent equilibrium constants are defined as:

$$K_e(DAI) = \frac{[HI\text{-}OR][H_2O]}{[DAI][Thr\text{-}OR]} = \frac{\alpha \times 0.555 \times \%H_2O}{(1-\alpha)[Thr\text{-}OR]}$$

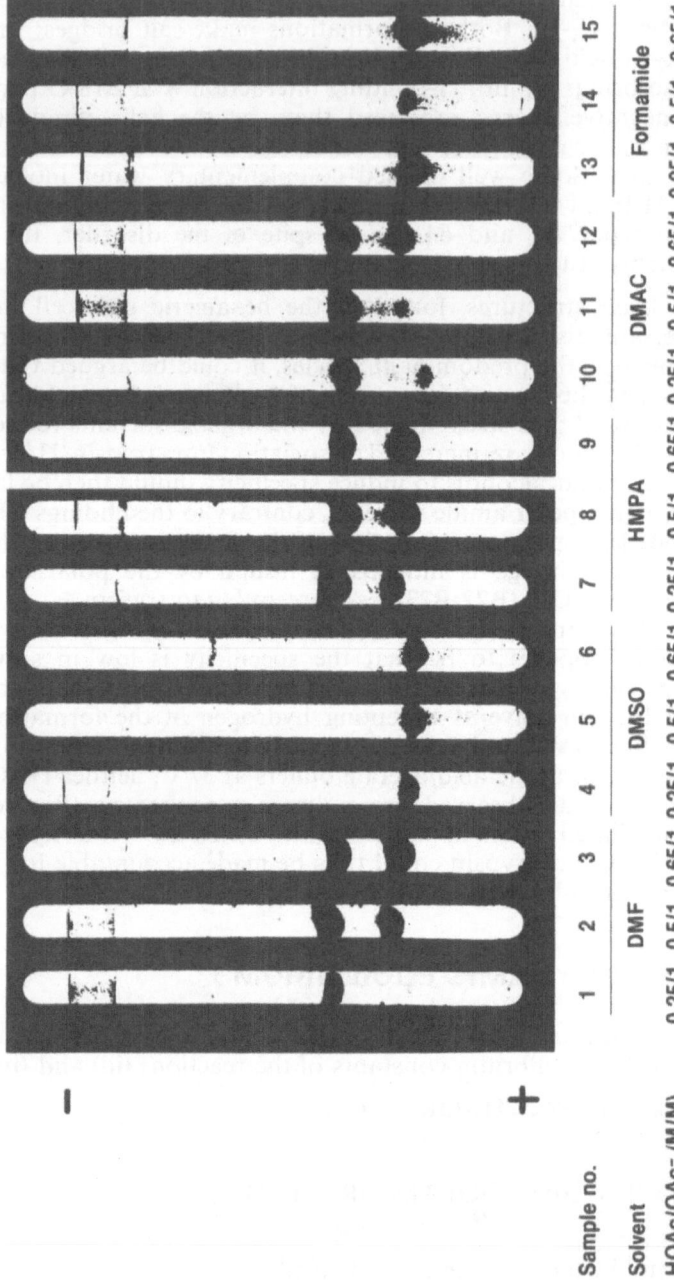

Figure 16 Disc electrophoretic analysis of yields in the conversion of porcine insulin to human insulin methyl ester in 43% H_2O in five organic solvents. For each solvent three levels of acidity, HOAc/OAc$^-$ = 0.25/1, 0.5/1 and 0.65/1, were tried. Temperature 37°C, sampling 24 h.

54

and

$$K_e(\text{DOI}) = \frac{[\text{DOI-Thr-OR}][\text{H}_2\text{O}]}{[\text{DOI}][\text{Thr-OR}]} = \frac{\beta_2 \times 0.555 \times \%\text{H}_2\text{O}}{\beta_1[\text{Thr-OR}]}$$

For each threonine ester equations (iii) and (iv) give rise to two equilibrium constants, one for the DAI equilibrium denoted by I and one for the DOI equilibrium denoted by D. The threonine esters are denoted by M (Thr-OMe), B (Thr(Bu^t)-OBu^t), SB (Thr-OBu^t), E (Thr-OEt), Tmb (Thr-OTmb) and Mse (Thr-O-(CH$_2$)$_2$-SO$_2$-CH$_3$). Combinations of I or D with threonine ester symbols unambiguously define the equilibrium constant, e.g.:

$$K_e(\text{DSB}) = \frac{[\text{DOI-Thr-OBu}^t][\text{H}_2\text{O}]}{[\text{DOI}][\text{Thr-OBu}^t]}$$

In a typical experiment using 1 M Thr-OMe and 20% water, 99% coupling yield, viz. $\alpha/(1 - \alpha) = 99$, corresponds to an equilibrium constant of 1100 and 90% coupling yield to a constant of 100. The problem in determining $K_e(\text{DAI})$ is the chromatographic separation of DAI from porcine insulin and, if Thr-OR is Thr-OMe, from human insulin formed by hydrolysis of HI-OMe during reaction and/or preparation for analysis. The problem with interference from porcine insulin can be circumvented if the equilibrium in equation (iii) is established using either DAI, human insulin, human insulin ester or single-chain des-(B30) insulin (SCI) as the starting material. Another point that requires caution is that DAI is usually determined as a peak of a few percent in a chromatogram, identified by its retention time only. Besides human insulin, other unforeseen by-products might be formed and accidentally coelute with DAI. If so $K_e(\text{DAI})$ is being underestimated. One such compound that coelutes with DAI is DOI-Thr-OBu^t. Two other identified compounds that either coelute or elute close to DAI are des(Phe^{B1})HI-OMe and Arg^{B0} HI-OMe, compounds formed by transpeptidation of the corresponding biosynthetic single-chain precursors B(2–29)-Ala-Ala-Lys-A(1–21) insulin and Arg-B(1–29)-Ala-Ala-Lys-A(1–21) insulin, both possible contaminants of the starting material, viz. B(1–29)-Ala-Ala-Lys-A(1–21) insulin (SCI-AAK).

A seemingly correct method to check the K_e value is to establish the equilibrium using two different threonine esters in equimolar ratios, e.g. Thr-OMe and Thr(Bu^t)-OBu^t each 0.5 M.

(v) $$K_e(\text{IM}) = \frac{\alpha[\text{H}_2\text{O}]}{(1 - \alpha)[\text{Thr-OMe}]}$$

(vi) $$K_e(\text{IB}) = \frac{\alpha_1[\text{H}_2\text{O}]}{(1 - \alpha_1)[\text{Thr(Bu}^t)\text{-OBu}^t]}$$

Since $1 - \alpha$ and $1 - \alpha_1$ both represent DAI, division results in

(vii) $$K_e(\text{IM})/K_e(\text{IB}) = \frac{\alpha}{\alpha_1}$$

If $K_e(\text{IB})$ is determined separately, $K_e(\text{IM})$ should be determinable from (vii).

Since HI(Bu^t)-OBu^t does not hydrolyse to HI, determination of DAI becomes unambiguous. However, a consequence of the kinetic model in Chapter 6 is that the K_e(IM)/K_e(IB) ratio depends upon the threonine ester mixture in the medium, the ratio being highest when calculated for equilibria where the threonine esters are separated. Furthermore, the activities of the threonine esters are not independent of each other in mixture, as proton transfer takes place from the weaker base (Thr-OMe) to the stronger base (Thr(Bu^t)-OBu^t).

The ratio between DOI-Thr-OR and DOI has been determined at the later stages of transpeptidation, where the main reaction (I) has been completed. Since DOI/DOI-Thr-OR formation continues as long as HI-OR is available, the ratio β_2/β_1 can be used to calculate K_e(DOI) if the equilibrium (iv) adjusts itself at a substantially higher rate than that by which new DOI and DOI-Thr-OR are being generated, most likely in another ratio than that of the equilibrium. The same argument applies to the ratio $\alpha/(1 - \alpha)$ when the SCI molecule is the substrate that feeds new molecules into the equilibrium (iii). As the coupling reaction (iii) is faster than transpeptidation reactions the use of the ratio $\alpha/(1 - \alpha)$ to estimate K_e(DAI) in a dynamic situation where substrates like SCI are still being converted is a justifiable approximation. Nevertheless, a direct measurement of K_e(DAI) using the fast coupling reaction (iii) is to be preferred.

Water and threonine esters are present in such large excesses that their concentrations can be regarded as being constant.

Table 32 illustrates an experiment where the problem of determining K_e(IM) is impeded by the simultaneous hydrolysis of HI-OMe to HI, which coelutes with DAI and is accounted for as such. Although coupling of DAI to HI-OMe is a fast reaction, transpeptidation of HI to HI-OMe is not. The accumulation of HI is therefore a function of trypsin concentration, and the K_e(IM) values appear to decrease with decreasing concentration of trypsin. From such an experiment K_e(IM) can be stated to be larger than the largest estimated value, K_e(IM) > 350.

In one case special precaution was taken to analyse the DAI in equilibrium without interference from either HI or PI (Table 33). First, human insulin was used as substrate in order to exclude porcine insulin in the DAI peak in the HPLC analysis. Secondly, the LiChrosorb RP-18 (5μ) column that can separate DAI and HI was applied for analysis of the samples at equilibrium after 144 h. Thirdly, the DAI peaks from the analytical column were collected, diluted with water, desalted by binding to Sep-Pak™ (Water Ass.) followed by wash with water, eluted with formic acid in 50% acetonitrile and, finally, evaporated to dryness. For details see Chapter 6, section 3. The samples of DAI thus recovered were analysed for N-terminal amino acids and for amino acid composition. Both analyses were in accordance with the theory for DAI, rendering the yields of DAI likely to be correctly assigned to DAI and not to unforeseen contaminants. A small amount of the DAI ($< 5\%$) is expected to be desamido-(A21) human insulin. The chromatogram of the experiment using 8 mM human insulin as substrate and sampled at 144 h is shown in Figure 8. The K_e(IM) values are calculated to range from 375 to 480, the variation being due to the sensitivity of K_e to small variations in the amounts of DAI, and not significantly correlated to insulin concentration.

Higher precision in the determination of K_e can be obtained at lower concentrations of threonine ester and higher concentrations of water; both means by which to increase the amounts of DAI in equilibrium (Table 34). Keeping the acid/base ratio constant at 1.5/1, K_e(IM) is found to be constant for concentrations of Thr-OMe varying between 0.5 and 0.063 M and for concentrations of water varying between 25 and 32%. Since K_e(IM) is constant, the effect of varying the water concentration in this narrow range is explained satisfactorily by the law of mass action applied to equation (iii). The greater part of the effect of water concentration on the dissociation of the carboxylic acids (see Chapter 1, equation (xii) and Homandberg et al.[14]) may occur at higher concentrations of water when the solvent is DMAC. A value of K_e(IM) of about 700 is estimated.

In a similar experiment the concentrations of acetic acid and acetate were kept constant at 1.5 and 1 M, respectively, but the equilibrium in 1 M Thr-OMe was compared to the equilibrium in 0.1 M Thr-OMe plus 0.9 M N-methyl morpholine (Table 35). The inhibitory action of Thr-OMe on transpeptidation prevents establishment of equilibrium in 1 M Thr-OMe within 24 h, whereas in 0.1 M Thr-OMe plus 0.9 M N-methyl morpholine a value for K_e(IM) of 550 is determined, in fair agreement with already mentioned results using DMAC as the organic solvent.

Coupling between DAI and Thr(Bu^t)-OBu^t (Table 36), proceeds more slowly than between DAI and Thr-OMe (Table 32). The apparent decrease in K_e(IB) with decreasing concentrations of trypsin in Table 36 reflects the lack of adjustment to equilibrium at the lower concentrations of trypsin. Values of K_e(IB) of about 400–430 were determined at the higher concentrations of trypsin.

Varying the insulin substrate concentration in solutions of Thr(Bu^t)-OBu^t leads to estimates of K_e(IB) of 300 both for coupling and transpeptidation (Table 37). The variation in K_e(IB) between experiments, cf. Tables 36 and 37, is larger than the standard deviations within an experiment, pointing to the difficulty in reproducing the experimental conditions precisely enough to avoid such large variations when a reactant (DAI) is present as a small percentage only.

The K_e(IM)/K_e(IB) ratio in Thr-OMe/Thr(Bu^t)-OBu^t 0.5/0.5 (M/M) mixture was determined to 1.22 ± 0.03 using insulin concentrations from 2 to 16 mM (Table 38). The experiment in Table 39 results in a similar ratio between equilibrium constants. However, the K_e(IM)/K_e(IB) ratio depends upon the ester mixture as demonstrated in Figure 17. With increasing amounts of Thr-OMe in Thr(Bu^t)-OBu^t, keeping the total concentration of threonine esters constant at 1 M, the ratio K_e(IM)/K_e(IB) increases. The finding is a combination of two types of interactions between the threonine esters, viz. a competition for binding to trypsin, cf. kinetic model in Chapter 6, and a proton exchange between threonine esters, Thr(Bu^t)-OBu^t being a stronger base than Thr-OMe (Table 1).

The estimate of 300 for K_e(IM) (Table 39) is in the lower end of the range in comparison with earlier estimates of about 400 (Table 33), about 700 (Table 34) and 550 (Table 35), all estimates at 12°C and using an acid/base

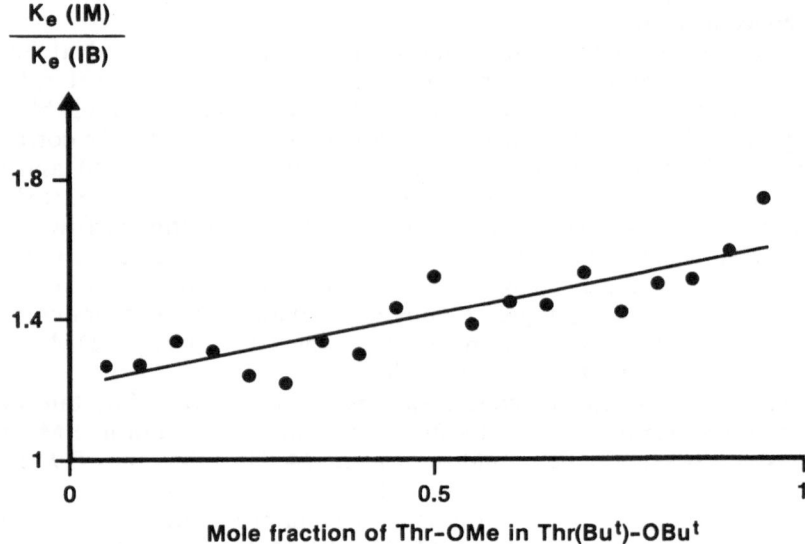

Figure 17 Ratio between equilibrium constants K_e(IM) and K_e(IB) as a function of Thr-OMe/Thr(Bu^t)-OBu^t ratio. Conditions: Thr-OR 1 M, acetic acid/acetate 1.5/1 (M/M), H_2O 20.7%, organic solvent DMAC and temperature 12°C

ratio of 1.5/1. Thus, in view of the variation in the determined values for the equilibrium constants, the best estimates are K_e(IM) = 500 $\pm$ 200 and K_e(IB) = 300 $\pm$ 150. Inouye et al.[108] reported values for K_{syn} = [R$_1$CO-NH-R$_2$]/[R$_1$COOH] [NH$_2$R$_2$] of about 50 in 20% water in both BD and DMSO/glycerol 1/1 for the coupling of Boc-Lys-OH to Val-OBu^t. If the K_{syn} value is converted to the equilibrium constant by multiplication with the molar concentration of water, a K_e value of about 550 is derived, in good agreement with the K_e(IM) and K_e(IB) values in DMAC in 20.7% water.

Attempts to reveal the correlations between the acidity in the medium and K_e(IM) are found in Tables 15 and 16. Due to the lack of precision and provisos involved in the determination of K_e(IM), no such correlation was established in the buffer range from H$^+$-Thr-OMe/Thr-OMe = 0.5/0.5 (M/M) to HOAc/OAc$^-$ = 1.5/1 (M/M). The temperature has too little effect on K_e values to enable the establishment of a correlation, cf. Tables 15, 18, 24, 26, 29, 40 and 42. Furthermore, at higher temperatures the determinations of K_e are complicated by enzyme inactivation, which may precede equilibrium.

Besides Thr-OMe and Thr(Bu^t)-OBu^t four other threonine esters were tested at 12°C at HOAc/OAc$^-$ ratios of 1.5/1 and 2/1, namely Thr-OEt, Thr-OMse, Thr-OBu^t and Thr-OTmb, Tables 21 and 41. In both experiments a long time was taken to ensure equilibrium, but in the experiment shown in Table 41 the SCI molecule is used as substrate. Since it is transpeptidized slowly to HI-OR in equilibrium with DAI, unconverted SCI is still present after 72 h in the presumed equilibrium between HI-OR and DAI. If a tentative ranking of threonine esters with respect to the corresponding K_e

values is permissible from these limited data, the ranking would be:

$$\text{Thr-OMe} > \text{Thr(Bu}^{\text{t}}\text{)-OBu}^{\text{t}} \geqslant \text{Thr-OMse} > \text{Thr-OTmb}$$

$$\geqslant \text{Thr-OEt} > \text{Thr-OBu}^{\text{t}}$$

As already shown by Inouye $et\ al.$[108], the type of solvent has a pronounced influence on the equilibrium constants. The strongly polar, aprotic solvents provide the highest equilibrium constants. This most probably means that the activity coefficients of water are more reduced in such solvents than in alcohols, ethers and ketones, conceivably by strong solvent–water hydrogen bonding. Table 24 shows comparisons of four solvents at three different concentrations of water. It is found consistently that:

$$K_e(\text{IM})\text{DMAC} \simeq K_e(\text{IM})\text{DMF} > K_e(\text{IM})\ \text{acetone}$$

A graduated decrease in K_e is found when DMAC is diluted with BD (Table 42). Though unconverted SCI is still present after 73 h, the slow transpeptidation of this molecule in comparison with the fast adjustment of the equilibrium justifies the estimation of K_e in the dynamic situation. Similarly, the K_e values are lower in DMSO/BD 1/1 than in DMAC (Table 43), whereas in DMSO/BD 4/1 the $K_e(\text{IM})$ could not be estimated since the insulin compounds partly fibrillated, cf. Table 44. In the ranking of solvents with respect to K_e, BD falls into the same group as acetone and THF, cf. Tables 26 and 24. The solids used as organic solvents, i.e. acetamide, polyethylene glycol and mixtures thereof, do not result in K_e values attractive for synthesis, cf. Tables 29–31. Finally, the data lend themselves to a comparison of $K_e(\text{I})$ versus $K_e(\text{D})$. It is a feature in most of the solvents that the $K_e(\text{I})$ are larger than the $K_e(\text{D})$ values, $vide$ Tables 24, 42 and 45. Only in solutions of acetamide and polyethylene glycol can the reverse be observed (Tables 29–31). As the equilibria that are being compared have adjusted in the same solution where the concentrations of water and threonine ester are in common, the choice of solvent influences the ratio of activity between insulin compounds:

$$\frac{K_e(\text{I})}{K_e(\text{D})} = \frac{a_{\text{HI-OR}} \times a_{\text{H}_2\text{O}}}{a_{\text{DAI}} \times a_{\text{Thr-OR}}} \times \frac{a_{\text{DOI}} \times a_{\text{Thr-OR}}}{a_{\text{DOI-Thr-OR}} \times a_{\text{H}_2\text{O}}}$$

$$= \frac{a_{\text{HI-OR}} \times a_{\text{DOI}}}{a_{\text{DAI}} \times a_{\text{DOI-Thr-OR}}}$$

It is likely that it is the activities of DAI and DOI that are prone to selective changes as a function of solvent, since the two different C-terminal basic amino acids of DAI and DOI might have additional degrees of freedom to change their potentials in different solvents, for example by salt-bridge or hydrogen bond formation, as compared to the possibilities in DAI-Thr-OR and DOI-Thr-OR.

In summary: the apparent equilibrium constant is constant, i.e. the activity coefficients are constant, in mixtures of water and DMAC at concentrations of water from 20% to 30%. Equilibrium constants are sufficiently high to secure more than 97% human insulin ester in equilibrium when using 1 M threonine ester and 20% water, corresponding to a change in free energy, ΔG_0, of about $-15\,kJ/mole$. The strongly polar, aprotic solvents are the most efficient to promote synthesis, namely to displace reaction (iii) to the right. Although a lower percentage of water can be applied in milder solvents, like BD, the equilibrium constant is more than correspondingly reduced, so it is recommended to use DMF or DMAC as the most efficient 'equilibrium displacement' solvents.

5. REACTION RATES

The reaction rate itself is unimportant for the yield and the economy of the process, as the homogeneous reaction in a small volume requires minimal investments, merely a vessel. Of importance, however, is the ratio between the reaction rate and the rate by which the trypsin is inactivated: in other words, yields decrease if the reaction rate is slowed down to such an extent that trypsin becomes inactivated before the equilibrium has been established. The measures taken to improve specificity, that is lower temperature, lower concentration of water and higher acidity in the medium, all have the effect of lowering the reaction rates. There is a limit to the acceptable slowness of the transpeptidation reaction, one particular problem being the physical stability of insulin in aqueous–organic solutions, as gels form with time, the so-called fibrillation.

The determination of the activation energy from the slope of ln$k$ versus $1/T$ (viii) in the Arrhenius plot is impeded by nonlinearity of such plots between 0 and 12°C.

(viii)
$$E_A = -R\frac{\Delta \ln k}{\Delta (1/T)}$$

The influence of increasing the temperature by 8°C in the range between 4 and 12°C is a doubling of reaction rates for both coupling and transpeptidation (Table 46), corresponding to activation energies of about 50 kJ/mole. But between 0 and 4°C the reaction rates also double, meaning activation energies of about 100 kJ/mole. As a consequence of the nonlinearity of the Arrhenius plots the estimations of activation energy for coupling and transpeptidation are not very accurate[71] (Table 46). However, as there is no significant difference between the activation energies of coupling and transpeptidation, the large difference in reaction rates cannot be accounted for in terms of activation energy. Between 12 and 21°C reaction rates are approximately doubled (Table 29), and between 12 and 25°C, using the SCI substrate, there is an increase in rate by a factor of 3.5–4 (Table 42). The moderate reduction of reaction rate by a factor 2 for 8°C is amply regained by the increase in trypsin stability by lowering the temperature, in particular between 25 and 8°C in the most acidic buffer (HOAc/OAc$^-$ = 1.5/1 (M/M); Table 5), where stability increases 15–20-fold by a decrease of 8°C. Consequently, it is advantageous to lower the temperature to well below the commonly used 37°C.

Increasing the acidity in the reaction medium from acetic acid/acetate = 1/1 to 1.5/1 (M/M) has a slight influence on reaction rates (Tables 15 and 29). In the acetic acid/acetate buffer range there is, however, a limit to how much acid is acceptable before reactions come to a stop, even with the fast coupling reactions (Table 47). Using an acetic acid to acetate ratio of 4/1 (M/M) coupling still proceeds, but at ratios 6/0.67 (M/M) and higher, reactions do not proceed at all. This means that the ratio between k and the stability of trypsin has a maximum somewhere in the acetic acid/acetate buffer range.

The reduction in water concentration at 12°C only has a modest effect on the stability of trypsin (Table 5). Below about 20% water in DMAC, reaction rates become so slow that several days are required to reach 90% conversion in transpeptidation reaction (Table 15). The ratio between reaction rate and trypsin inactivation rate will increase with increasing concentrations of water and has no optimum in the operational range. It is the demands for specificity and equilibrium displacement that set the upper limit for the water concentration.

In practice reaction times necessary to ensure 99% conversion (7 half-lives) may vary from less than half an hour in coupling reactions to several days in transpeptidation reactions, dependent upon trypsin concentration.

6. COUNTER ANIONS

The anions produced when the threonine ester is neutralized with an acid should be strong enough bases to accept protons from the protonated form of the threonine ester, and thus be able to release the amino group for its nucleophile attack on the acyl-enzyme. Hence anions of strong acids like hydrochloric acid and phosphoric acid should be avoided. The point is illustrated in Tables 48–50. Yields are reduced if half the threonine ester is neutralized with HCl, and the use of 1 equivalent of HCl results in virtually no conversion (Table 48). If a buffer system of pyridinium chloride/pyridine 0.9/0.9 (M/M) is used in connection with 0.5 M threonine ester the hydrochloric acid is transferred from the weaker base (pyridine) to the stronger base (threonine ester) and, therefore, reaction is prevented (Table 49 and Figure 18). Reactions proceed in pyridinium acetate. Likewise reaction can proceed if half an equivalent of phosphoric acid is added to the threonine ester, whereas with one equivalent reaction is abolished (Table 50). The specificity is low in the buffer having half an equivalent of phosphate in this solvent which is acetamide. Jonczyk and Gattner[73] reported inhibition of transpeptidation at Arg^{B22} in phosphate buffers in 60% DMF, stating that the specificity was provided by the phosphate ions. The apparent inconsistency might well be explained by the different solvents used. Formic acid is also too strong an acid to permit reaction, and the use of 1.25 equivalents of formic acid relative to the threonine ester completely abolishes reaction (Table 50). Remaining useful acids to neutralize the threonine esters are the weak carboxylic acids, preferably acetic acid.

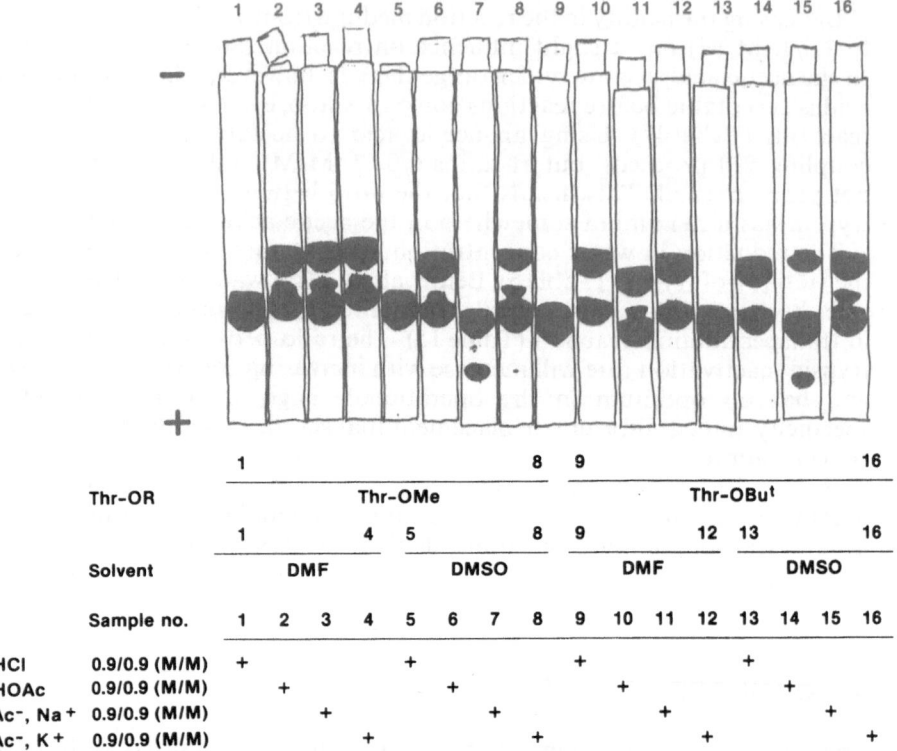

Figure 18 Disc electrophoresis of samples from coupling reactions. Coupling of DAI to human insulin methyl ester (samples 1–8) and of DAI to human insulin *t*-butyl ester (samples 9–16). Sampling after 24 h at 37°C. The evaluation of yields and conditions is shown in Table 49. The gels Nos. 1, 5, 9 and 13 are analyses of samples buffered with pyridinium chloride/pyridine, demonstrating complete inhibition of coupling due to transfer of HCl from the weaker base (pyridine) to the stronger base (threonine methyl ester)

7. INSULIN SUBSTRATES

A variety of insulin compounds were transpeptidized to human insulin methyl ester. The compounds were porcine proinsulin (Table 51 and Figure 19) and in another experiment Arg^{B31}-Arg^{B32} porcine insulin, rabbit insulin (Ser^{B30} porcine insulin), and a mixture of des(Arg^{31}-Arg^{32}) porcine proinsulin and des(Lys^{62}-Arg^{63}) porcine proinsulin (Table 52). Apparently proinsulin is transpeptidized in better yields than porcine insulin and Arg^{B31}-Arg^{B32} porcine insulin in better yields than rabbit insulin, suggesting that prolongations beyond residue B30 increase reaction rates due to a lowering of K_m caused by bindings to the subsites S'_2 and S'_3 of trypsin. Figure 19 shows the result of the first transpeptidation experiment in organic solvents, November 12, 1979.

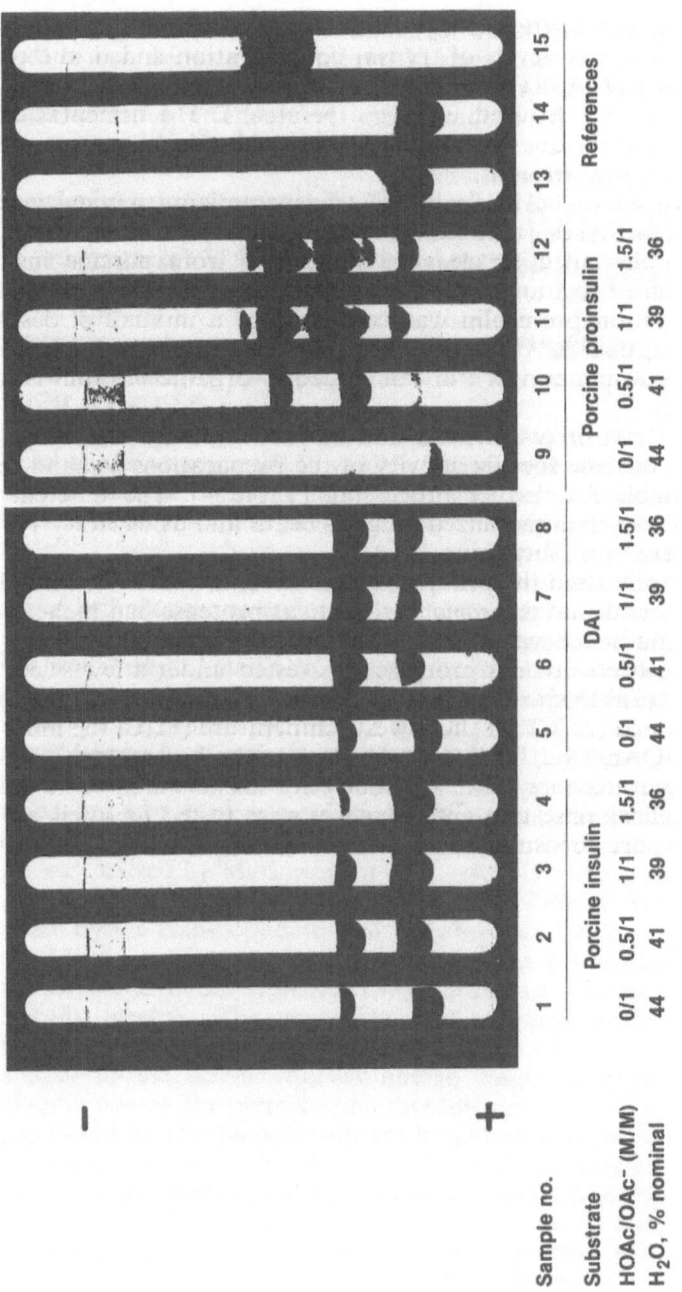

Figure 19 Disc electrophoretic analysis of the first transpeptidation experiment. Substrates: gels 1–4 porcine insulin; gels 5–8 DAI; gels 9–12 porcine proinsulin. References: gels 13–14 porcine insulin, gel 15 porcine proinsulin. The estimated yields are shown in Table 51. Conditions: temperature 37°C; organic solvent DMF; %H$_2$O and HOAc/OAc$^-$ as indicated below figures.

Sample no.	1	2	3	4	5	6	7	8	9	10	11	12	13	14	15
Substrate	Porcine insulin				DAI				Porcine proinsulin				References		
HOAc/OAc$^-$ (M/M)	0/1	0.5/1	1/1	1.5/1	0/1	0.5/1	1/1	1.5/1	0/1	0.5/1	1/1	1.5/1			
H$_2$O, % nominal	44	41	39	36	44	41	39	36	44	41	39	36			

8. ENZYMES

Two batches of TPCK-treated trypsin and three different grades of trypsin were compared at two levels of trypsin concentration and in the presence and absence of EDTA (Table 53). No significant difference between trypsin preparations can be deduced from the results. The detrimental effect of EDTA is most likely due to binding of residual calcium ions originating from the trypsin preparations.

Plasmin proved to be incapable of transpeptidizing porcine insulin to human insulin methyl ester (Table 54), in accordance with earlier experiments in which plasmin failed to cleave alanine B30 from porcine insulin[112]. Plasmin also failed to transpeptidize porcine proinsulin (Table 54), whereas in aqueous solution proinsulin was converted to a mixture of des(Ala^{B30}) insulin and des(Ala^{B30}), Arg^{A0} insulin[112]. A straightforward explanation of the failure of plasmin to work in this aqueous–organic medium is its lack of stability.

Immobilized trypsin works, but the amounts required to bring about synthesis with the low specific activity of the preparations at hand resulted in gels unsuitable for further processing (Table 54). The different yields obtained with trypsin immobilized on glass beads and using either Thr-OMe or Thr-OBu^t are most surprising.

Morihara[84] discussed the problem of low specific activity of immobilized enzymes and found that *Achromobacter lyticus* protease had higher activity than trypsin and hence was a better candidate for immobilization.

The *Achromobacter lyticus* protease was tested under a few selected sets of conditions (Table 55). The best yields were obtained at the highest temperature tested (25°C). At the lowest temperature (12°C) the most acidic buffer, HOAc/OAc,⁻ 1.2/1.2 (M/M), resulted in the best yields.

Finally, three enzymes with specificity for basic amino acid residues, streptokinase, urokinase and enterokinase, were tested for their ability to transpeptidize porcine insulin. In no case could such activity be demonstrated (Table 56).

5
Conversion of single-chain insulin precursors into human insulin esters

1. EARLIER STUDIES

During the search for enzymes that would cleave proinsulins to a limited extent only, Markussen[112] found that porcine plasmin was a suitable candidate. Two main products were produced, des(Ala^{B30}) insulin and Arg^{A0},des(Ala^{B30}) insulin; cleavage of the Arg^{B22}-Gly^{B23} bond was not observed. In the same study, by an elaborate and ambiguous semisynthetic route involving affinity chromatography on immobilized insulin antibodies, 50 μg of the single-chain B(1–29)-A(1–21) insulin precursor (SCI) was obtained. It was suggested that this molecule could be the product of fermentation, and be used as an insulin precursor – when genetic engineering became a reality some time in the future – because it was shown to possess two important properties. Firstly, that the molecule after a reduction could be reoxidized in fair yields (> 50%) similar to proinsulin and, secondly, that it could be cleaved with plasmin between Lys^{B29} and Gly^{A1} rendering des-(Ala^{B30}) insulin, a fully potent insulin derivative.

The topic was revived by Markussen et al.[86], when it was found that the molecule could be synthesized from porcine insulin in DMAC-water by an intramolecular tryptic transpeptidation in the absence of threonine esters. Having access to the compound in substantial amounts it was found that it could be crystallized as rhombohedra similar to insulin and that the molecule was biologically inactive. The mere fact that it could be formed by transpeptidation implied that it should be possible to open up the single-chain precursor to the double-chained human insulin ester by tryptic transpeptidation, now in the presence of a threonine ester.

The key question of how the molecule could fold up and recover after a redox cycle, was reinvestigated by Markussen[87], this time varying pH and temperature. Although optimum conditions found for good recovery in these *in vitro* experiments are far from conditions *in vivo* as far as temperature, pH, and the lack of a protein: thiol-oxidoreductase are concerned, the SCI molecule was always recovered after a redox cycle in higher yields than porcine proinsulin. In the assessment of yields use was made of HPLC; hence SCI and proinsulin could be reduced and oxidized together, making possible a comparison of recoveries under truly identical conditions.

The finding that the reduced form of the SCI molecule was able to fold in such a way that the correct disulphide bridges of insulin were formed by oxidation suggested that the (SCI) molecule could be produced by genetic engineering. Consequently, the corresponding gene was synthesized by site specific mutagenesis, inserted in a plasmid and expressed in yeast.[88] Another advantage of the SCI molecule as compared to proinsulin was the absence of pairs of basic amino acids, potential enzymatic cleavage sites in yeast since maturation of the yeast pheromone, the α-factor, implies cleavages at Lys-Arg residues[113]. Attempts to express human proinsulins in yeast resulted in the appearance of C-peptide in the fermentation broth, and yields of proinsulin were correspondingly low[88]. In the expression of the SCI molecule in yeast use was made of this enzymatic activity to achieve cleavage between the leader sequence and the Phe^{B1} residue of SCI, the result being expression and secretion of mature SCI.

2. HYDROLYSIS OF SINGLE-CHAIN INSULIN PRECURSORS BY PLASMIN

The early study on cleavage of SCI by plasmin[112] was carried out using 2 nmol of SCI and identifying the cleavage between Lys^{B29}-Gly^{A1} by a positive dansyl-glycine. Since glycine could have been detected as false positive, the cleavage reactions were repeated using SCI and SCI-AAK as substrates and HPLC to monitor the conversions. A Tris buffer of pH 8.25 and an acetate buffer of pH 5.5, both containing 0.01 M lysine for plasmin stabilization, were used for the digestions at 37°C. The results appear in Table 57.

The HPLC diagrams revealed that some degradation to desoctapeptide-(B23–B30) insulin had taken place, for plasmin an unexpected cleavage at the Arg^{B22}-Gly^{B23} sequence (Figure 20). Information was then acquired that plasminogen usually is activated by trypsin, and that a trypsin contamination of about 1% remains in the plasmin product. The experiments were repeated using urokinase activated plasminogen. The plasmin prepared by urokinase activation of plasminogen was incapable of cleaving SCI-AAK (Figure 20). Thus, it appears that the originally proposed strategy for biosynthesis of des(Ala^{B30}) insulin[112] by plasmin cleavage of the Lys^{B29}-Gly^{A1} bond of SCI is impracticable, and that the observed cleavage was due to the contaminating trypsin. The yields of DAI obtained as a result of the contaminating trypsin are quite high (Table 57), and a workable strategy having a step of limited tryptic hydrolysis of SCI, yielding DAI, followed by coupling with a threonine ester in organic–aqueous medium could be envisaged. However, a one-step tryptic transpeptidation of the single-chain insulin precursor to human insulin esters appeared more attractive.

3. TRANSPEPTIDATION OF SCI TO HI-OR USING TRYPSIN

Using, at first, the semisynthetic SCI(ss)[86] that became available June, 1983, it was found that the Lys^{B29}-Gly^{A1} bond of SCI was far less prone to cleavage

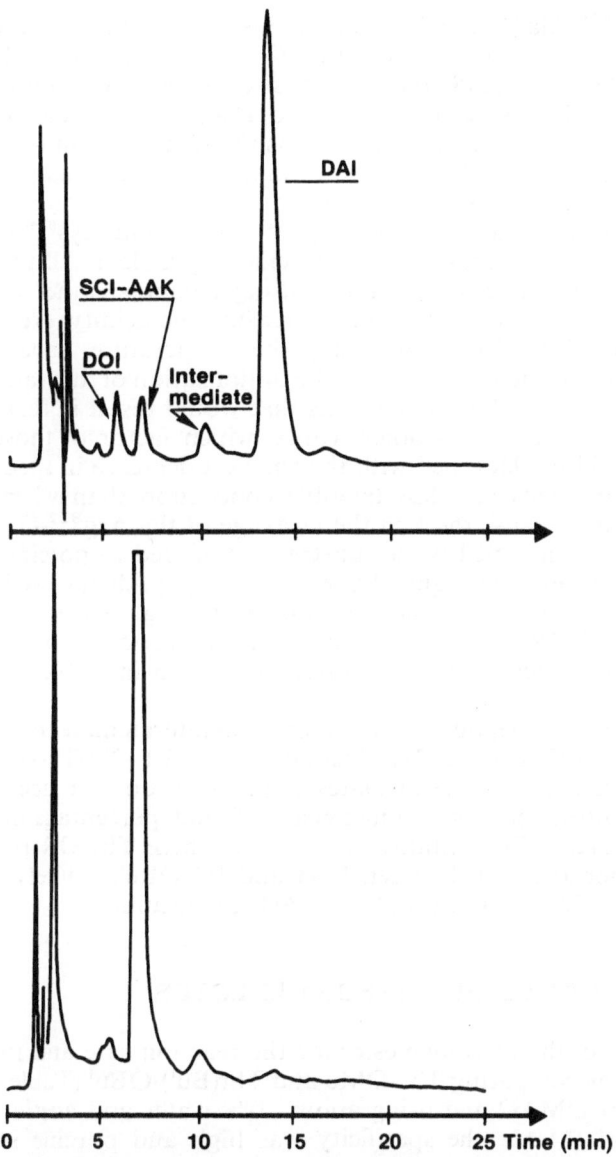

Figure 20 Top: Cleavage of single-chain insulin precursor, SCI-AAK, to DAI by trypsin activated plasmin. Digestion 72 h at 37°C in Tris buffer pH 8.25, cf. Table 57. Note beside unsymmetrical peak of intermediate(s) a by-product formation of DOI, a cleavage caused by contaminating trypsin. Bottom: same experiment using urokinase activated plasminogen

than the Lys^{B29}-Ala^{B30} bond of porcine insulin. Using the standardized set of conditions of 20.7% water in DMAC, acetic acid/acetate 1.5/1 (M/M), 1 M Thr-OMe, and 0.2 mM trypsin, a first-order rate constant of $0.0068\,h^{-1}$ was found for the conversion of SCI to HI-OMe. For the conversion of porcine insulin under the same conditions the rate constant was found to be $0.18\,h^{-1}$. The joining of the carboxyl terminal of the B-chain with the amino terminal of the A-chain apparently introduces a steric hindrance making the two trypsin susceptible sites, viz. Arg^{B22}-Gly^{B23} and Lys^{B29}-Gly^{A1}, much alike, and thereby emphasizing the specificity problem. All the changes in factors known to increase k, namely using alcohols rather than DMAC, increasing the water concentration, decreasing the acidity, exchanging Thr-OMe with $Thr(Bu^t)$-OBu^t and raising the temperature, have the effect of decreasing the specificity. The aim of the optimization of the transpeptidation of SCI became a search for conditions that would result in reasonably high k and specificity values: in other words, which factor of those known to increase k could be slackened with the smallest decrease in specificity as the result. The specificity is a less tangible conception than when converting porcine insulin, because the k in the cleavage of the Arg^{B22}-Gly^{B23} bond is largely reduced when SCI is the substrate compared to porcine insulin and DAI as substrates. Consequently, when transpeptidizing SCI, DOI plus DOI-Thr-OR formation is slow in the beginning, but when substantial amounts of HI-OR have been formed, the by-product formation speeds up. Examples of such reaction progress are shown in Tables 42, 45, 62, 63 and 64.

When SCI is transpeptidized, two additional intermediates can be foreseen, viz. B(1–22)/B(23–29)-A(1–21) insulin and B(1–22)-Thr-OR/B(23–29)-A(1–21) insulin. These intermediates apparently do not accumulate, but small, unidentified and unaccounted peaks of small percentage may represent such intermediates. For instance, in the case where Thr-OR is Thr-OBu^t a peak is temporarily seen between DAI and HI-OBu^t, a likely position for elution of B(1–22)-Thr-OBu^t/B(23–29)-A(1–21) insulin.

4. SIGNIFICANCE OF THREONINE ESTER

The influence of the threonine ester for the reaction rate and the specificity is illustrated by comparing Thr-OMe and $Thr(Bu^t)$-OBu^t (Tables 43 and 58). In the solvent DMAC and using about 20% water and acetic acid/acetate equal to 1.5/1 (M/M), the specificity was high and porcine insulin could easily be converted to HI-OR using either threonine ester. Using SCI as substrate, formation of HI-OMe is strongly inhibited, whereas formation of $Hi(Bu^t)$-OBu^t proceeds at reasonable rate and with a specificity so high that yields approaching 90% are obtained (Tables 43 and 58). If the acidity is decreased from acetic acid/acetate 1.5/1 to 0/1 (M/M), formation of HI-OMe can take place, whereas in $Thr(Bu^t)$-OBu^t the specificity is lost and DOI-$Thr(Bu^t)$-OBu^t becomes the major product (Table 58). If the solvent DMAC is exchanged with DMSO/BD 1/1 (v/v) and the acidity is retained at acetic acid/acetate concentrations of 1.5/1 (M/M), the rate of formation of HI-OMe increases, whereas the rate of formation of HI(Bu^t)-OBu^t decreases (Tables 43 and 58). An explanation of this adverse behaviour could be that Thr-OMe inhibits transpeptidation by strong binding to the S_1' site of trypsin and thereby prevents binding of insulin substrates, whereas Thr(Bu^t)-OBu^t binds less firmly. A change in conditions that loosens binding of Thr-OMe to trypsin increases k because the acyl-enzyme formation is the rate determining step. In Thr(Bu^t)-OBu^t, where acyl-enzyme formation is not necessarily the rate determining step, not only is a decrease in reaction rate observed when DMAC is exchanged with DMSO/BD, but once again, the specificity is lost, as indicated by heavy formation of DOI-Thr(Bu^t)-OBu^t. The inhibition of transpeptidation of porcine insulin by Thr-OMe has been reported earlier[70,71] and is further treated in Chapter 6. Discrepancies in rates between experiments, cf. Tables 43 and 58, are largely due to variations of the water concentration within the narrow range of importance, variations difficult to reduce in the small scale experiments.

In conclusion, one way to achieve high yields in transpeptidation of SCI to HI-OR is to choose Thr(Bu^t)-OBu^t as the threonine ester, DMAC as solvent, a water concentration about 20% and maintain a ratio of acetic acid/acetate of 1.5/1 (M/M).

Thr-OBu^t has properties between those of Thr(Bu^t)-OBu^t and Thr-OMe and it was consequently used as a probe to evaluate a variety of solvents and mixtures of solvents.

5. RATING SOLVENTS

At a constant concentration of water of 22.3%, the k for conversion of SCI to HI-OBu^t increases through the series of aprotic, polar solvents diluted with 10% BD (Table 59):

$$DMAC < DMSO < DMF < acetone$$

The specificity increased through the series

$$Acetone < DMF < DMSO < DMAC$$

The same series is obtained if the solvents have been diluted with 19% BD, and the water concentration reduced to 20% (Table 60). In acetone and t-butanol the specificity is inadequately low. DMF and DMAC appear to be equivalent in specificity but quite different with respect to k, in that 5 and 24 h data in DMF are similar to 24 and 48 h data in DMAC, respectively. So k values in 20% H$_2$O in acetic acid/acetate 1.5/1 (M/M) can be improved from the 0.0068 h^{-1} using Thr-OMe in DMAC to 0.03 h^{-1} using Thr-OBu^t in 19% BD in DMAC, or to about 0.02 h^{-1} in DMAC (Tables 60 and 61).

The use of mixtures of BD and DMSO was recommended by Rose et al.[75]; a series of experiments were conducted using such mixtures (Tables 44 and 64), as well as a series of experiments using mixtures of BD and DMAC (Tables 42, 45, 61–63). In the whole range of mixtures of DMAC/BD from 0/1 to 1/0 (v/v), and using an acetic acid/acetate ratio of 1.5/1 (M/M), there is no or very little variation in k as a function of variation in the DMAC/BD ratio, both when using Thr(Bu^t)-OBu^t (Table 42) and Thr-OBu^t (Tables 45, 61–63). The specificity drops markedly with increasing amounts of BD in the mixtures, the conclusion being that BD should be avoided. Similarly, no or very little effect on k values found for reactions in various DMSO/BD mixtures using acetic acid/acetate 1.5/1 (M/M) and 1 M Thr/OMe, whereas the specificity drops markedly with increasing BD concentrations (Tables 44 and 64). In DMSO there appears to be trypsin inactivation even at 12°C, and in DMSO/BD 4/1 (v/v) inactivation is observed at 25°C (Table 44). Consequently, also DMSO and mixtures of it with BD were abandoned as suitable solvents for transpeptidation of SCI to HI-OR, thus leaving DMF and DMAC as the preferred solvents.

6. THE ACIDITY FACTOR

The acidity could be reduced from the often used ratio of 1.5/1 (M/M) for acetic acid/acetate down to 0/1, with some gain in k but without loss of specificity, provided the organic solvent is DMF or DMAC and the threonine ester is Thr-OMe or Thr-OBu^t. The k for converting SCI to HI-OMe in DMAC in 20.7% H_2O increased from 0.0068 h^{-1} in acetic acid/acetate 1.5/1 (M/M) to 0.011 h^{-1} when this ratio was reduced to 0/1 (Table 58). Similarly, for the conversion of SCI to HI-OBu^t in DMF, reaction rates could be demonstrated to increase without concomitant loss of specificity by reducing the acetic acid/acetate molar ratio from 1.14/1.14 to 0/1.14 (Table 65) or from 0.28/1.14 to 0/1.14 (Table 66). The only exception to the rule, the example having 20.0% water and an acetic acid/acetate molar ratio of 0.28/1.14 of Table 66, is explained by an erroneously high content of water as revealed by the Karl Fischer analysis. Consequently, equimolar amounts of Thr-OR base and acetic acid, or equivalently, the acetate salt of the threonine ester without addition of acetic acid, were applied in the final optimizations.

7. WATER CONCENTRATION

For the two very similar solvents, DMF and DMAC, different concentrations of water result in the optimal yields. Both rate and specificity depend critically upon the water concentration being within very narrow limits, viz. less than 1% H_2O. The importance of the water concentration for k is shown in Table 67. For a decrease of 1% water the k values are reduced by a factor of about 2.

The Karl Fischer analysis of water content in reaction mixtures was included in order to verify the actual concentrations, realizing that the reproducibility of the final concentration of water, brought about in a total of 350–400 μl by micropipetting 3–4 additions of solvents, is no better than 7–8% of the water content, viz. about 1.5% of the nominal percentage of water. The optimization of water concentration in DMF was performed using 1.14 M Thr-OBu^t hydroacetate at 12°C. The optimum is between 21 and 22% H_2O nominal, analysed to be between 21.2 and 22.6% H_2O by the Karl Fischer method (Tables 65, 66 and 68). The attainable yield of 85–

90% is the same with different concentrations of trypsin, but the maximum appears earlier using the higher trypsin concentration (Table 68). The difference in optimal water concentration using either DMF or DMAC appears to be 2–3% in the transpeptidation of the SCI-AAK precursor to HI-OMe, DMF being the 'milder' solvent for trypsin, in which the lowest water concentration is optimal (compare Tables 72 and 73 with Table 75).

8. OTHER ENZYMES THAN TRYPSIN

Morihara et al.[81] used A. lyticus protease at 37°C in coupling of DAI and Thr-OBu^t to make HI-OBu^t. The lysine specific A. lyticus protease was able to transpeptidize SCI to HI-OMe in 26% water in DMSO/BD 1/1 (v/v) (Table 69). Reactions were slow too when using this enzyme, but in contrast to trypsin the higher temperature, 25°C, is advantageous as compared to 12°C, indicating a less progressive autolysis with increasing temperature for the A. lyticus protease. In another experiment, the A. lyticus protease was studied in DMAC at neutral and acid conditions using 21.4% and 28.6% water (Table 70). In this solvent the best yields were obtained at neutral conditions and at the lowest water concentrations.

Succinylated trypsin is most active using acidic conditions. No product is formed from SCI and Thr-OMe in 21.4% H_2O in DMAC under neutral conditions, whereas HI-OMe is formed in 28.6% water in DMAC using an acetic acid/acetate ratio of 1.67/1.11 (M/M) (Table 70). Succinylated trypsin also works in DMSO/BD 1/1 (v/v) in acetic acid/acetate 1.5/1 (M/M) (Table 69), whereas the activity is abolished in acetic acid/acetate 0.125/1 (M/M) in DMAC and 19.8% water (Table 71). So it appears as if succinylation of trypsin has changed the activity maximum in organic–aqueous media towards more acidic conditions. If the results in Tables 69 and 58 are compared, it appears that succinylated trypsin and bovine trypsin cleave less specifically than porcine trypsin in DMSO/BD 1/1 (v/v), 19.7% water, using acetic acid/acetate in a molar ratio of 1.5/1 at 12°C.

9. OTHER SUBSTRATES, SCI-SK AND SCI-AAK

On the basis of the hypothesis that the sluggishness of the transpeptidation of SCI to HI-OR was due to steric hindrance at the Lys^{B29}-Gly^{A1} cleavage site, genes were constructed for two new SCI analogues, having extensions of 2 and 3 amino acids between Lys^{B29} and Gly^{A1}, viz. genes coding for Ser-Lys and Ala-Ala-Lys insertions[88]. The corresponding products SCI-SK and SCI-AAK were expressed in yeast, extracted from the broth and purified chromatographically. The transpeptidation experiments are compiled in Tables 72–75.

Since two sites have to be cleaved, viz. Lys^{B29}-X^{B30} and Lys^{A0}-Gly^{A1}, two intermediates as well as their hydrolysis products are to be expected. New temporary peaks were observed in various positions, but since there was no build-up of intermediate products it is presumed that the opening of the single peptide chain renders the second site more disposed for cleavage than in the intact single chain. The HPLC chromatogram of the components in a conversion of SCI-AAK to HI-OMe featuring intermediate products is shown in Figure 21. The third intermediate peak is clearly inhomogeneous, indicating the presence of at least two components. At a later stage these intermediate peaks disappear. In one case, the transpeptidation of SCI-SK in Thr-OMe, substantial amounts of a suspected intermediate were observed (Table 72).

The hypothesis of a steric hindrance being the cause of the slow transpeptidation of SCI proved to be correct, as both SCI analogues were transpeptidized at higher rates than SCI. The order of the rates was:

$$SCI\text{-}SK > SCI\text{-}AAK > SCI$$

This order is valid using Thr-OMe as well as Thr-OBu^t, independent of the acidity in the medium (Table 72). In the calculation of first-order rate constants, an overall rate constant covering both cleavages has been assessed for the prolonged SCI analogues in order to allow a direct comparison of efficacy. On average, the rate constant increases by a factor of 2.6 by changing

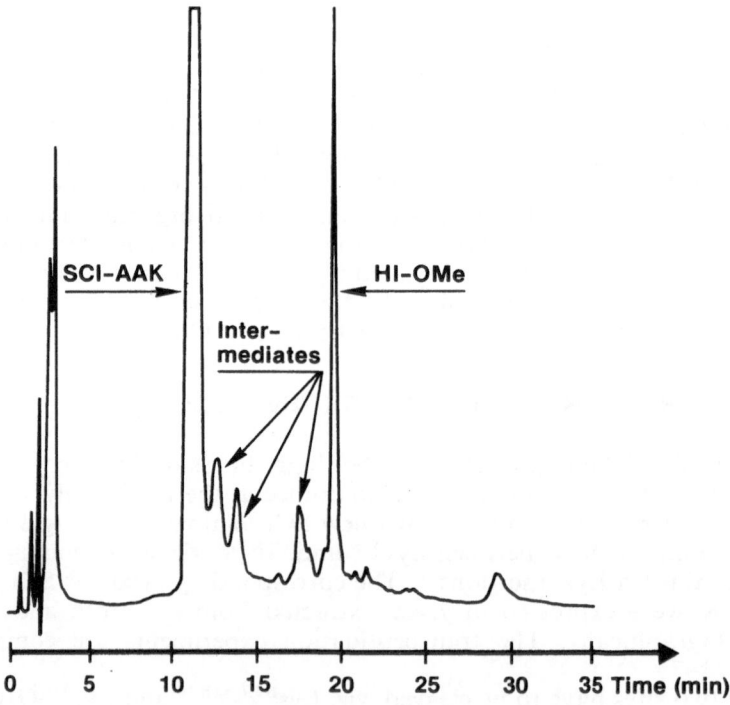

Figure 21 HPLC of transpeptidation of crude SCI-AAK to HI-OMe by trypsin. Besides starting material and product unknown, temporary peaks appear, most likely the foreseeable intermediates. Conditions: 5 mM SCI-AAK dissolved in 21% H_2O in DMF; 1 M Thr-OMe; acetic acid/acetate 1.5/1 (M/M); temperature 12°C; 0.2 mM porcine trypsin and 3 mM Ca^{2+}. Sampling 3.5 h. Gradient elution

from SCI to SCI-AAK and by another factor of 2.6 by changing from SCI-AAK to SCI-SK; the average being taken over the four experiments with each substrate.

An alternative explanation for the sluggishness in transpeptidation of SCI, namely that the Lys-Gly sequence binds poorly to trypsin, can be refuted since the substrates more accessible to cleavage contain the same sequence.

From Table 72 it can be deduced that the shift from acetic acid/acetate 1.7/1.14 (M/M) buffer to the 0/1.14 (M/M) buffer on average increases k by a factor of about 3, and that the shift from Thr-OMe to Thr-OBu^t increases k by a factor of 2.6. Yields approaching 90% conversion in the transpeptidation of SCI-AAK in 21% H_2O in DMF in acetic acid/acetate 0/1.14 (M/M) buffer could be achieved within 72 h even when the trypsin concentration was reduced to one third (Table 73).

Another way to increase the initial rate when transpeptidizing SCI-AAK in Thr-OMe is to reduce the concentration of Thr-OMe (Table 74). This inhibitory effect of Thr-OMe was also demonstrated in the transpeptidation of porcine insulin to HI-OMe (cf. Table 35). In the long run the yields do not improve by the reduction in concentration of Thr-OMe, despite the increase in initial rates, mainly due to a small decrease in specificity (Table 74).

Finally, the water concentration was optimized in DMAC using an acetic acid/acetate buffer of 0/1.14 (M/M) (Table 75). The optimum found at about nominal 22.4–23.4% H_2O, corresponding to 22.5–22.9% in the Karl Fischer analysis, is a small percentage higher than the optimum in DMF (cf. Tables 72 and 73). The pure solvents, both Fluka puriss, p.a., were found by Karl Fischer analysis to be virtually free of water, viz. <0.1%. Hence it can be concluded that DMAC per volume is the most powerful solvent of the two with respect to ability to induce specificity and to decrease the reaction rate of tryptic transpeptidations in the useful water concentration range from 20 to 25%.

In summary: biosynthetically produced single-chain precursors featuring a bridge from Lys^{B29} to Gly^{A1} can be transpeptidized by trypsin in the presence of threonine esters yielding human insulin esters. The preferred conditions are: organic solvent DMF or DMAC; water concentration 20–25%; acetic acid 1 equivalent relative to threonine ester when using Thr-OMe and 2.5 equivalent when using Thr(Bu^t)-OBu^t. If Lys^{B29} is bound direct to Gly^{A1}, transpeptidation is slow, presumably due to steric hindrance. Consequently, cleavage at Arg^{B22} causes major by-product formation. At all sets of conditions, the threonine esters can be ranked with respect to rate of transpeptidation as follows:

$$\text{Thr(Bu}^t\text{)-OBu}^t > \text{Thr-OBu}^t > \text{Thr-OMe}$$

Two additional single-chain insulin precursors, featuring Ser-Lys and Ala-Ala-Lys bridges between Lys^{B29} and Gly^{A1}, were transpeptidized to human insulin esters. At all sets of conditions, the ranking of transpeptidation according to rate is:

$$\text{SCI-Ser-Lys} > \text{SCI-Ala-Ala-Lys} > \text{SCI}$$

Obviously, the incorporation of additional amino acids in the bridge has reduced the steric hindrance.

Manufacture of human insulin, by fermentation in yeast of a single-chain precursor followed by transpeptidation to a human insulin ester, commenced January 12, 1987 at the Novo plant in Kalundborg.

6
Kinetic studies

1. MODEL AND CONDITIONS

The kinetics of the interconversion of five insulins were studied at a standardized set of conditions. The five insulin compounds were des-(B30) insulin (I), porcine insulin (IA), human insulin (IThr), human insulin methyl ester (IM) and human insulin $Thr^{B30}(Bu^t)$-OBu^t (IB). A diagram of the reactions is shown in Figure 22. Concentrations of water, Thr-OMe, $Thr(Bu^t)$-OBu^t, trypsin, and acyl-enzyme are denoted by W, M, B, T, and IT. Michaelis–Menten complexes are shown with a comma between insulin and trypsin. T denotes free trypsin and T[0, W, M, B] denotes trypsin associated with either nothing (0), water (W), Thr-OMe (M), or $Thr(Bu^t)$-OBu^t (B).

The standardized conditions were: the concentration of threonine ester 1 M, the acetic acid/acetate ratio 1.5/1 (M/M), the nominal percentage of water 20.7, the organic solvent DMAC and the temperature 12°C. Karl Fischer water analysis showed a water content of $21.3 \pm 0.7\%$ (SD). Finally, the system comprised 3 mM Ca^{2+} for stabilization of trypsin. One reason for the selection of these conditions is that trypsin is so stable that its concentration can be considered constant during the first 6 h of observation, cf. Chapter 4, section 2. In this solution initial inactivation for 0.2 mM trypsin is about 1% per hour at 12°C. Another reason for the selection of these conditions is that the large value of the equilibrium constants for the synthesis of human insulin esters from des-(B30) insulin enables the use of data until 35% conversion in the calculation of forward first-order rate constants (k values) without interference from the reverse reactions.

Kinetic data of some of the reactions in Figure 22 using the same set of conditions have been reported earlier[70,71], and computer simulation of reaction progress curves was attempted[71]. The pronounced inhibition exerted by Thr-OMe on transpeptidation of porcine insulin was treated as a direct inhibition of the release of alanine from the transition state, according to the hypothesis due to a firm binding of Thr-OMe to His^{46} of the active site of trypsin. The consequence of that model was that rate constants for reactions leading from Michaelis–Menten complexes to the acyl-enzyme varied with the type of threonine ester in the medium. Supplementary and revised experimental data will be given in this chapter. Furthermore, a new model is proposed, in which the inhibitory action of Thr-OMe on transpeptidation

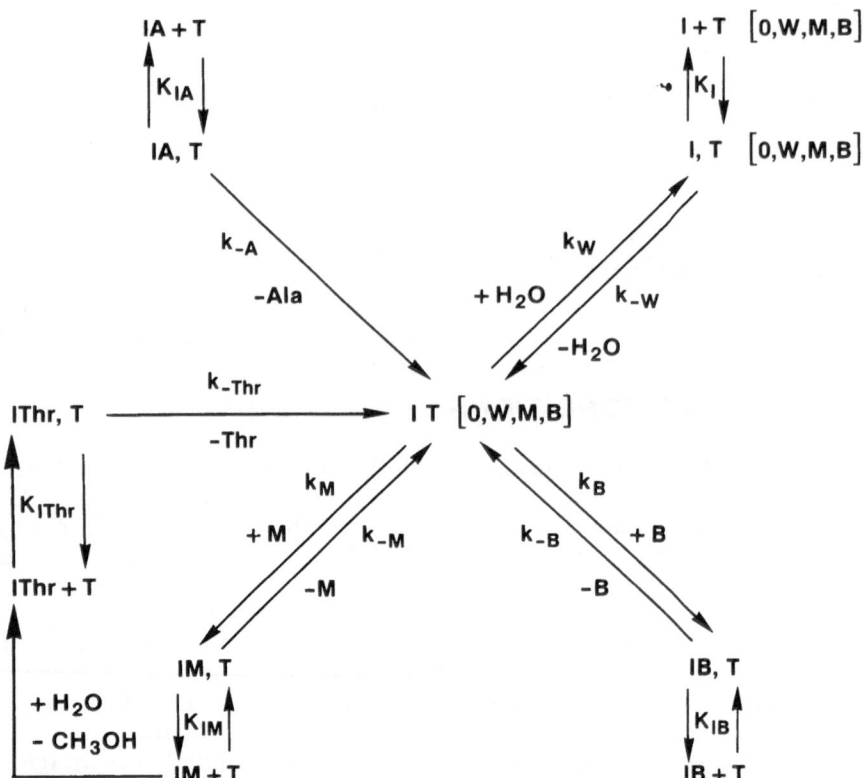

Figure 22   Reaction diagram of reactions in kinetic study. Symbols are: IA: porcine insulin; I: des-(B30) insulin; IM: HI-OMe; IB: HI(Bu^t)-OBu^t; IThr: human insulin; T: trypsin; K_I, K_{IA}, K_{IM}, and K_{IB}: equilibrium dissociation constants; k_{-A}, k_{-W}, k_{-M}, and k_{-B}: rate constants leading to acyl-enzyme IT; k_M, k_B, and k_W: rate constants for aminolysis and hydrolysis of acyl-enzyme. W, M, and B denote water, Thr-OMe, and Thr(Bu^t)-OBu^t, and 0 denotes the absence of any of these three ligands

is treated as an example of competitive inhibition by the second substrate, meaning that insulin–trypsin binding is affected by the choice of threonine ester. Rate constants leading to acyl-enzyme (k_2) become independent of the threonine ester, a feature that renders the interpretation of resulting constants, derived by computer simulated curve fitting, more comprehensible than the constants of the earlier model.

The model, proposing competitive inhibition by binding of the second substrate, viz. the nucleophile, in the subsite S$'_1$, is in agreement with recent mechanistic studies on serine proteases[19,20]. Binding of water to acyl-trypsins prior to hydrolysis was proposed by Seydoux et al.[114]. Riechmann and Kasche[20] interpreted the inability of an amino component to completely inhibit hydrolysis as being due to different, non-overlapping S$'_1$ binding sites. In the present model competition between water and amino component for the same S$'_1$ subsite is presumed. However, if trypsin features a distinguished subsite for water, the reactions can still be simulated by the model, simply by making the trypsin–water dissociation constant large in comparison to the trypsin–amino component dissociation constant.

The monitoring of kinetic experiments by manual sampling and subsequent analysis of samples is not precise when reactions are fast, as in the coupling reactions. Consequently, coupling reactions were studied using smaller trypsin concentrations than the usual 0.2 mM used for transpeptidation. In order to enable a comparison between rate constants they have been normalized to 1 mM trypsin.

2. INITIAL VELOCITIES

First-order k values were estimated by linear regression analysis of $-\ln(S/100)$ vs. time, where S represents the percentage of unconverted substrate. Good correlations were retained for up to 35% conversion. Initial velocities, as expressed by k values, were proportional to enzyme concentrations. This is usually the rule, deviations from which must be explained by an inhibitor or an activator present in the enzyme preparation. A series of determinations of k values from different experiments using the same standard conditions are compiled in Table 76. The standard deviations are typically $\pm 10\%$ for transpeptidations and ± 25–30% for coupling reactions. The large standard deviations in the coupling reactions reflect the difficulty in monitoring fast reactions by the manual method. As there is no significant difference between the normalized k values either at different trypsin concentrations or at different substrate concentrations, a gross mean has been calculated for each reaction. Plots of $-\ln(S/100)$ vs. time cut the y-axis close to the origin and are evenly distributed around $y = 0$, meaning that initial bursts were insignificantly small. The values in Table 76 have been normalized to 1 mM trypsin to facilitate comparisons.

The fastest reactions are coupling reactions in 1 M Thr-OMe or in 0.5 M Thr-OMe plus 0.5 M Thr(Bu^t)-OBu^t, the k values being insignificantly different. Coupling between I and Thr(Bu^t)-OBu^t proceeds significantly slower than couplings in the presence of Thr-OMe, namely at about half the rate. The ranking of the transpeptidation reactions according to k values is:

$$IM \rightarrow IB \gg IA \rightarrow IB > IA \rightarrow IM > IThr \rightarrow IM$$

$$\gg IB \rightarrow IM$$

The inhibitory action Thr-OMe exerts on transpeptidation has been discussed earlier[70,71] (see also Table 35), and is apparent from this series. Note that porcine insulin is transpeptidized faster to human insulin methyl ester than human insulin meaning either that alanine is a better leaving group than threonine or that IA binds better to trypsin than IThr. On the other hand, Thr-OMe is an exceptionally good leaving group, and the transpeptidation rate of IM approaches that of coupling reactions. Thr(Bu^t)-OBu^t is apparently the least willing leaving group and this, in combination with the inhibitory effect of Thr-OMe, makes the IB $\rightarrow$ IM process the slowest encountered. However, this process is anomalous as will be discussed later.

The k values for transpeptidation or cleavage of porcine insulin analysed by amino acid analysis of alanine are shown in Table 77. For the reaction IA → IM there is a close coincidence of the mean values determined by HPLC of insulin compounds and by amino acid analysis, cf. Tables 76 and 77. For the IA → IB reaction the alanine formation precedes the IM formation slightly but significantly, indicating transitional accumulation of I. The ranking of amines with respect to k values for release of alanine is:

$$\text{Thr(Bu}^t\text{)-OBu}^t > \text{NMM} > \text{N(CH}_3)_4\text{-OH} > \text{Thr-OMe} > \text{N(Et)}_3$$

Once again the inhibitory action of Thr-OMe as compared to Thr(Bu^t)-OBu^t is demonstrated. Triethylamine or an impurity therein tends to irreversibly inhibit trypsin as the reaction comes to a stop before completion, earlier when using an old, opened bottle of N(Et)$_3$ than a fresh bottle.

Two dynamic relations between formation of components were obtained from kinetic studies during the initial phases of reaction. First, the ratio between formation of IM and IB in a mixture of Thr-OMe and Thr(Bu^t)-OBu^t, each 0.5 M, was determined to be 10/1, both when using IA as substrate (Table 38) and, more accurately, when using I as substrate and reduced concentrations of enzyme (Figure 23). Secondly, the ratio between formation of I and IB in the initial phases of the conversion of IM to IB could be determined. The initial I to IB ratio was earlier reported[71] to be 0.6/1. As the coupling of I to IB is rather fast (see Table 76), this ratio was underestimated due to late sampling. The ratio between I and IB formation in the initial phase is rather 2.5/1 as can be inferred from Figure 24. Both dynamic relations provide bonds between the rate and equilibrium constants shown in Figure 22, useful for the computer simulation of reaction progress.

Initial velocities (V_0) are for all reactions proportional to substrate concentrations (S_0) except for the IB → IM reaction. Lineweaver-Burk plots result in lines that cut through the origin, rendering the determination of K_m values impossible. This circumstance was discussed earlier[71], where a minimum value for K_m of 0.1 M was estimated for the IA → IM reaction. The Lineweaver-Burk plots for the other reactions are shown in Figures 25 and 26. None of the plots allows for an estimation of K_m. The dissociation between insulin compound and trypsin is large in the organic medium, and a further increase in substrate concentration above 8 mM is impractical as solutions become very viscous. In the computer simulations all the equilibrium dissociation constants between insulin compounds and trypsin (K_I, K_{IA}, K_{IM} and K_{IB}) were fixed at 0.1 M, viz. equal to the minimum estimate of K_m. By increasing the concentration of DMSO Fink[115] observed an exponential increase in K_m and a decrease in k_{cat} proportional to the decrease in water concentration in the α-chymotrypsin catalysed hydrolysis of N-acetyl-L-tryptophan p-nitrophenyl ester. In a study of the hydrolytic action of immobilized α-chymotrypsin, Tanizawa and Bender[116] reported an increase in K_m, a decrease in deacylation rate constant (k_3), and an invariable acylation rate constant (k_2) at increasing concentrations of dioxan. Likewise, in a study on peptide synthesis using immobilized α-chymotrypsin, N-acetyl amino acid esters as acyl donors and amino acid amides as amino components, Nilsson and Mosbach[117] found a large increase in K_m by changing the medium from

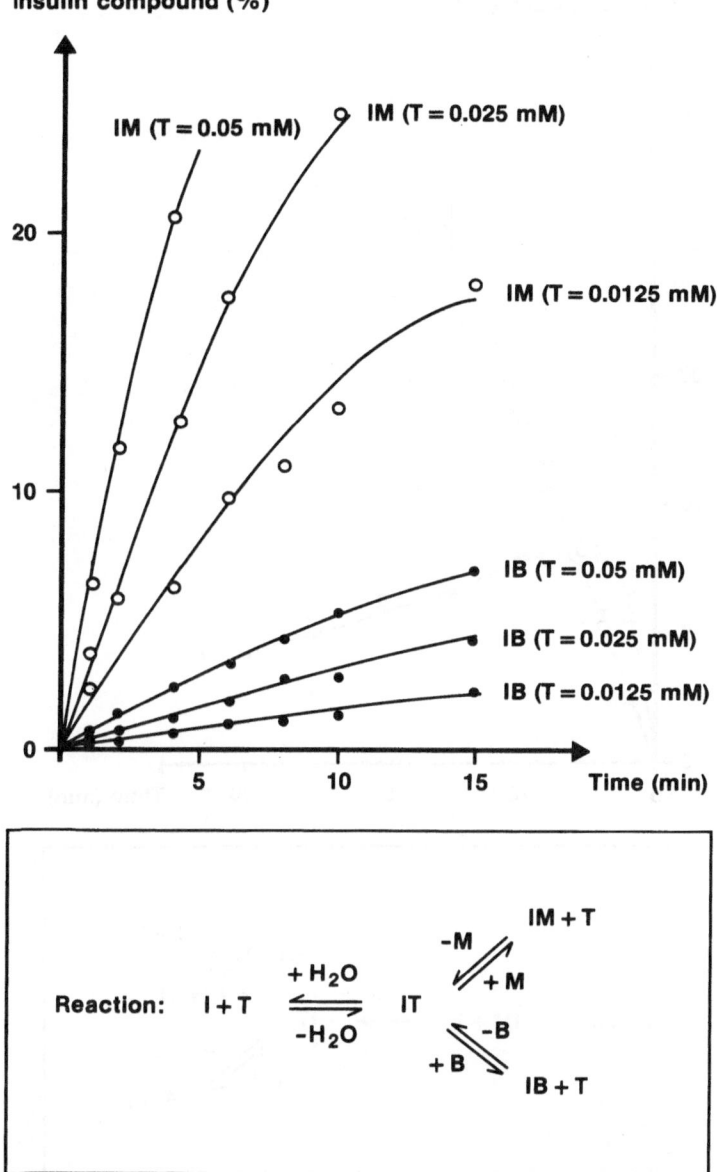

Figure 23 Formation of HI-OMe and HI(Bu^t)-OBu^t in mixtures of Thr-OMe and Thr(Bu^t)-OBu^t during initial stages of coupling reactions, using DAI as substrate. Independent of trypsin concentration the initial value of dIM/dIB is found to be 10. Standard conditions

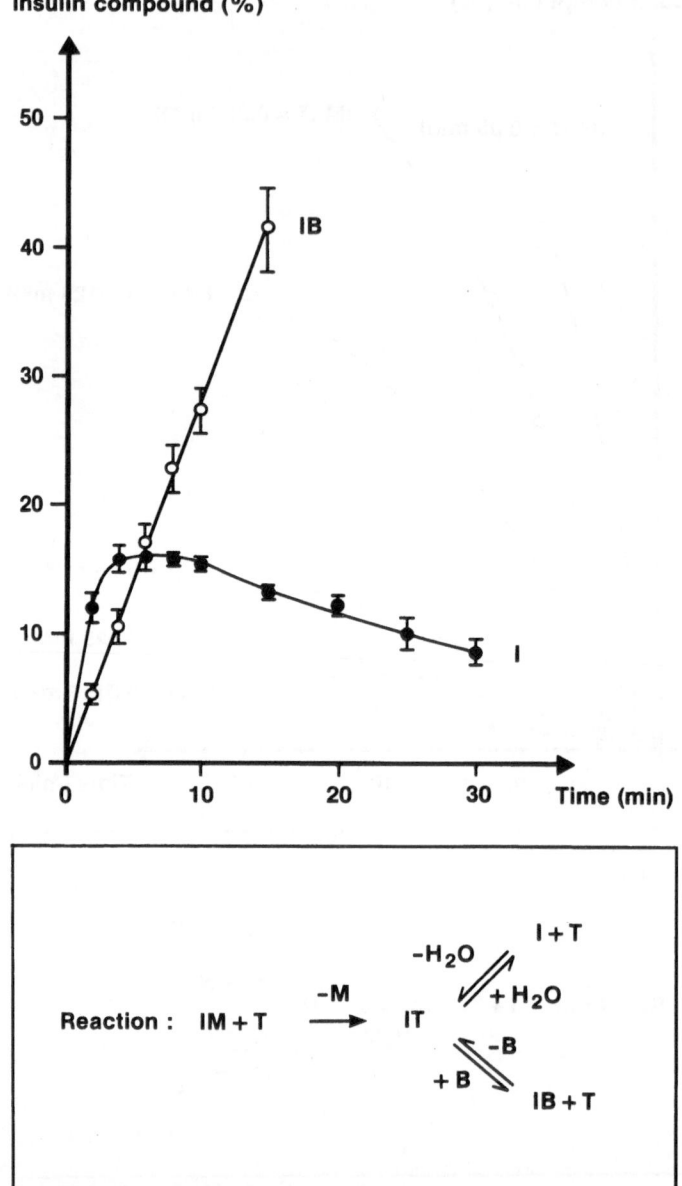

Figure 24 Transpeptidation of HI-OMe to HI(Bu^t)-OBu^t showing a transient peak of DAI. The initial value of dI/dIB is estimated to be 2.5. Standard conditions

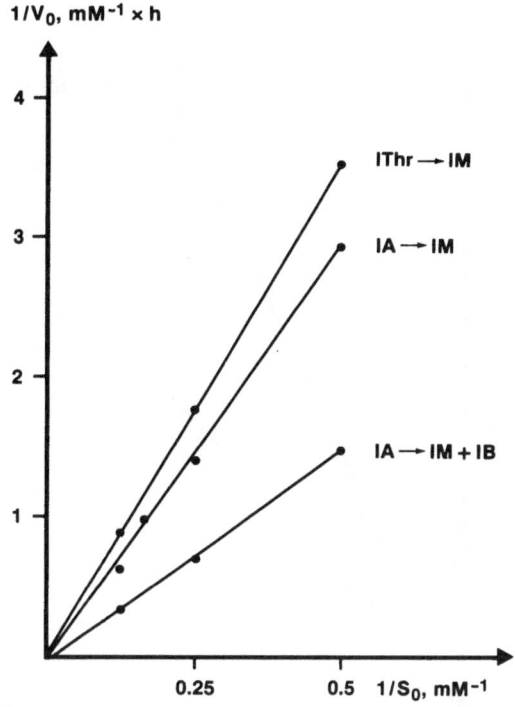

Figure 25 Lineweaver-Burk plots of three transpeptidation reactions, porcine insulin → HI-OMe, porcine insulin to a mixture of HI-OMe and HI(Bu^t)-OBu^t and human insulin → human insulin methyl ester. Standard conditions. The intercept with the abscissa equals $-1/K_m$ in this plot, but intercepts are too close to the origin to enable the estimation of K_m values

water to 50% DMF. Thus, the indeterminable, large K_m values at the selected standard conditions of the present studies are in agreement with the trends observed for chymotrypsin, viz. that organic solvents impair substrate binding.

The transpeptidation of IB to IM is anomalous in that the initial velocity increases with decreasing concentration of substrate. The plots of V_0 versus S_0 are shown in Figure 27. HI(Bu^t)-OBu^t is a very hydrophobic molecule and it could be envisioned that part of the decrease in V_0 with increasing S_0 could be due to associations between IB molecules, if such dimers were inaccessible to trypsin. The mixed syntheses of IM and IB resulted in a constant ratio of IM over IB of 1.22 independent of concentration of insulin compounds (see Table 38), indicating that if association between IB molecules occurs it is effective even at the lowest concentration of insulin compound. Another possibility was that the procedure, in which IB is dissolved in 10 M acetic acid and then mixed with Thr-OMe dissolved in DMAC, could produce t-butyl acetate, which eventually destroyed the active site of trypsin by alkylation. However, by mixing the components in reverse order, viz. dissolving IB in the final mixture comprising 1 M Thr(Bu^t)-OBu^t, DMAC and the acetic acid/acetate 1.5/1 (M/M) buffer resulted in a V_0 that varied

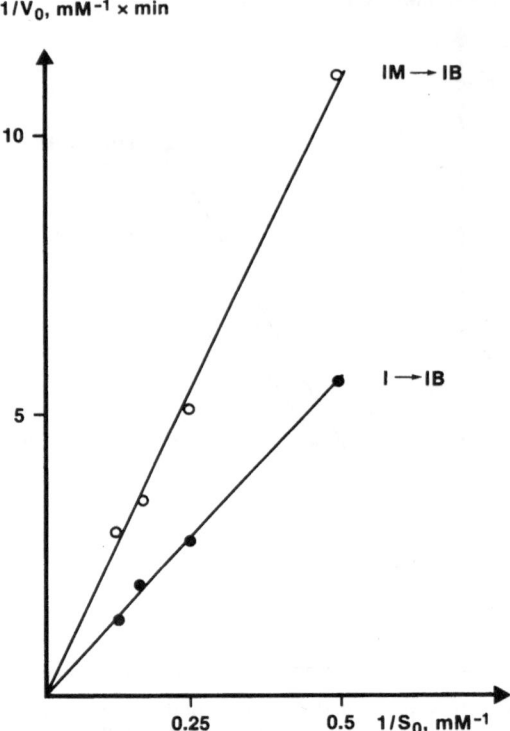

Figure 26 Lineweaver-Burk plot of transpeptidation reaction, HI-OMe → HI(Bu^t)-OBu^t, and of coupling reaction, DAI → HI(Bu^t)-OBu^t. Standard conditions. The intercepts with the abscissa are too close to the origin to enable the estimation of K_m values

insignificantly with S_0 (Figure 27). As no inhibition was observed during synthesis of IB from I, the inhibitory effect cannot be ascribed to IB itself, but rather to an inhibitor present in the solid preparation of HI(Bu^t)-OBu^t. An irreversible trypsin inactivation was subsequently demonstrated directly using the method described in Chapter 2, section 10. Within 10 min the amidase activity of the trypsin in 8 mM HI(Bu^t)-OBu^t was reduced to 50% of that in 8 mM porcine insulin, using the standardized conditions for the kinetic study. The most likely explanation of this inactivation appears to be a t-butylation of the active site of trypsin by a reactive molecule formed in the solid preparation of HI(Bu^t)-OBu^t during storage. It can be inferred from the computer simulation studies, using constants that provide for a fair simulation of the other processes, that the uninhibited conversion of IB to IM should progress somewhat slower than the conversion of IA to IM (compare Figures 30 and 33).

The hypothesis that the inhibition of transpeptidation by Thr-OMe is brought about by binding of Thr-OMe to the S$'_1$ site of trypsin cannot be refuted from what is known about the influence of the P$'_1$ residue on k_{cat}/K_m for synthetic substrates[118-120]. Liem and Scheraga[118] observed a 5-fold

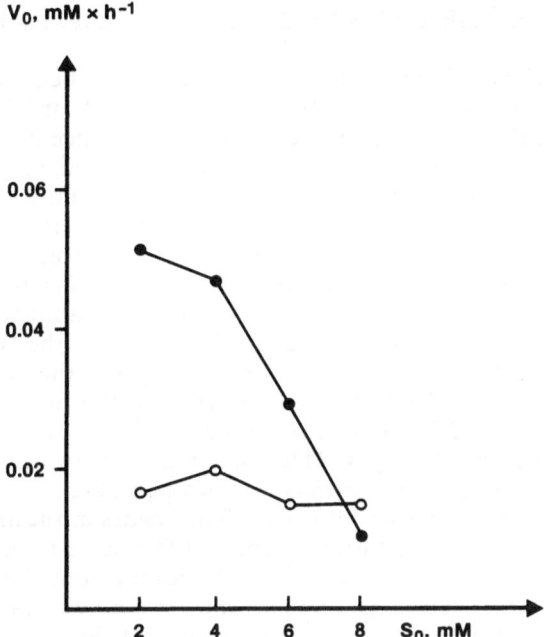

Figure 27 Plot of reaction rate in mM/h as a function of substrate concentration for the transpeptidation of HI(Bu^t)-OBu^t to HI-OMe using two different orders of adding the solvents. The anomalous behaviour indicates the presence of a trypsin inhibitor in the substrate. ●: dissolution of IB in 10 M HOAc; ○: dissolution of IB in buffer

increase in k_{cat} when P$_1'$ was changed from Gly to Ala in the substrate Gly-Val-Arg-Gly-NH$_2$. A further 10-fold increase in k_{cat}/K_m was achieved by changing Ala to Leu in the P$_1'$ position, indicating an affinity for a non-polar residue in the S$_1'$ site. Lobo et al.[119] found a 4–5-fold decrease in k_{cat}/K_m when Gly in position P$_1'$ was changed to Val in the peptide Ac-Arg-Gly-OMe. The combined results of the studies[118, 119] point towards the importance of steric fit between P$_1'$ and S$_1'$. Likewise, using thioester substrates of the type Boc-Arg-S-R, McRae et al.[120] found increasing k_{cat}/K_m values through the series:

Boc-Arg-SBu-i(Val analogue) < Boc-Arg-SPe-s(Ile analogue)

< Boc-Arg-SPe-i(Leu analogue)

In the light of these data and the Thr-OMe/Thr(Bu^t)-OBu^t findings, the following rule for fitting into the S$_1'$ site can be deduced: branching at the β-carbon of P$_1'$ leads to decreased binding if both branches are non-polar as in Val and Thr(Bu^t)OBu^t in comparison with branching where one branch is polar, as in Thr-OMe.

3. FLUXES IN THE DYNAMIC EQUILIBRIUM I ⇌ IM

The same equilibrium between I and IM is attained when the threonine ester is Thr-OMe, no matter whether the substrate is I, IA or IThr. Knowing the k for the I → IM reaction and the equilibrium concentration of I in the mixture, the flux of molecules through I can be assessed, provided the trypsin still has its initial activity at the time when equilibrium is established.

The equilibrium was studied using IThr as substrate rather than IA, because I and IThr can be separated by HPLC (see Figure 8). In the equilibrium attained the $K_e(IM) = (IM \times W)/(I \times M)$ was found to be independent of the concentration of insulin compounds, as expected (Table 33). In the I ⇌ IM equilibrium $2.7 \pm 0.4\%$ of the two insulin compounds is present as I, des-(B30) insulin. Using the best estimate for $k/T = 1.19\,min^{-1}\,mM^{-1}$ for the I → IM reaction the flux per hour through I equals $60 \times 1.19 \times 2.7\%$ per mM trypsin. Using 0.2 mM trypsin the flux is 38% per hour or 900% per 24 h, meaning that an insulin molecule on average passes through the I variety 9 times per 24 h.

A non-enzymatic hydrolysis of IM to IThr occurs in the medium, viz. ester hydrolysis, and the human insulin formed, IThr, is in turn, transpeptidized back to IM. From the rate equations in equilibrium the first-order rate constant for hydrolysis of IM to IThr can be derived. Using equation (ii), Chapter 2 and the second-order rate constant for trypsin autolysis of $0.055\,mM^{-1}\,h^{-1}$, as determined for the actual conditions, the residual trypsin concentration at 144 h can be derived to be 0.077 mM when starting with 0.2 mM. The first-order rate constant for ester hydrolysis k_h equals $(IThr/IM) \times k(IThr \to IM) \times T = 0.04 \times 0.0118 \times 0.077\,min^{-1} = 36 \times 10^{-6}\,min^{-1} = 0.002\,h^{-1}$, using the value of IThr/IM = 4% (Table 33). The actual loss as human insulin during the synthesis of human insulin methyl ester is thus dependent upon the trypsin concentration at the time the synthesis is stopped. Assuming 0.2 mM trypsin this loss amounts to 1.5%.

In accordance with equation (xxviii), Chapter 1, the flux through I of on average 9 times per 24 h is inconsistent with the ^{17}O-NMR study[69], in which no labelling of human insulin ester with ^{17}O during either coupling or transpeptidation could be demonstrated using the same conditions of synthesis. The conclusion from the ^{17}O-NMR study could be false if (a) the purchased $H_2{}^{17}O$ by mistake was $H_2{}^{18}O$ or $H_2{}^{16}O$, (b) the NMR instrument had failed, or (c) if trypsin could discriminate against hydrolysis with $H_2{}^{17}O$, a very unlikely isotope effect. The kinetic argument could be proven wrong, if the 2.7% I, identified by its retention time in HPLC analysis only, was a by-product eluting in this position. Care was taken to secure that the peak identified as I (see Figure 8) was in fact des-(B30) insulin. The eluate from the analytical column containing the I peak was collected from four runs of 0.5 mg each of NaCl/HCl precipitated insulin compounds. The combined eluates were diluted with 1 volume of water and applied at a rate of 1 ml/min to a Waters Sep-Pak™ C18 cartridge, previously rinsed with 50% CH_3CN followed by 0.05 M formic acid. After adsorption salts were removed by washings with 0.05 M formic acid and the adsorbed insulin was finally eluted with 1.5 ml 0.05 M formic acid in 50% acetonitrile. The eluate was evaporated to dryness and contained an estimated $50\,\mu g$. The amino acid composition of the product was determined by a Beckman 121 MB amino acid analyser after a standard hydrolysis at $110°C$ for 24 h using $40\,\mu g$ (6 nmole) of the product and $100\,\mu l$ 6 N HCl. The composition was in perfect accordance with the theory for des-(B30) insulin. The remaining $10\,\mu g$ was subjected to 10 cycles of Edman degradation using the Applied Biosystems 470A Protein Sequencer. The first 10 residues from the A- and B-chains (except cysteines) were found as expected from the sequences. The first cycle revealed the PTH derivatives of glycine (A1) and phenylalanine (B1) and no other major peaks of PTH amino acids. It was concluded that the peak presumed to be des-(B30) insulin by its retention time had been correctly assigned.

Having proved the correct assignment of the I peak, it could be argued that the 2.7% I found could arise from IT, viz. acyl-enzyme being hydrolysed during work up for analysis. In the most concentrated insulin solutions (8 mM) the molar ratio between trypsin and insulin is 0.2/8 = 2.5%, so, in all experiments the peak I could be accounted for as hydrolysed IT. However, if this was the case, the I/IM ratio would vary with insulin concentrations since the trypsin concentration is constant. Since the I/IM ratio was found to be constant when the insulin concentration was varied (Table 33), it must be concluded that a substantial part of the des-(B30) insulin cannot be derived from the acyl-enzyme IT.

Finally, the 2.7% I could in theory arise from residual tryptic activity in the 1 M acetic acid, in which the samples are dissolved for analysis. However, in 1 M acetic acid the pH is 2.4, sufficiently low to secure total trypsin inactivation. Since the ^{17}O-NMR study is also inconsistent with the study by Rose et al.[76], using $H_2^{18}O$ and mass-spectrometry, different conditions in the medium and another threonine ester, it is found likely that the inconsistency, although not located, is due to an error in the ^{17}O-NMR study.

4. SIMULATING THE PROGRESS OF REACTIONS

A first requirement to any model that simulates reaction progress is that the marked characteristics of the reactions can be imitated by fitting the variables. Of such characteristics to be simulated, we have:

(a) the transient peak of I in the IM → IB reaction,

(b) the transient peak of IM in the I → IM + IB reaction,

(c) the close to identical growth of Ala and IM in the IA → IM reaction,

(d) the gap between Ala and IB in the IA → IB reaction.

The attained equilibria, I ⇌ IM and I ⇌ IB must be simulated as well as the equilibrium in the mixed threonine esters, I ⇌ IM ⇌ IB. Furthermore, the model must account for the inhibitory effect of Thr-OMe on transpeptidation reactions. The model must simulate all reactions within the experimental errors. Finally, it is considered a must that the model to be proposed complies with the Michaelis–Menten concept and the theory of an acyl-enzyme intermediate commonly accepted for serine proteases.

The model to be proposed does not attempt to explain the inconsistency between ^{17}O-NMR data and kinetic data, but will rely on the kinetic evidence. Likewise no attempts have been made to accommodate the inactivation of trypsin in the IB → IM reaction in the model.

Let the concentrations of unassociated compounds be denoted by:

T : trypsin
I   : des-(B30) insulin
IA : porcine insulin, Ala^{B30}-insulin
IM: Thr^{B30}-OMe insulin
IB : Thr^{B30}(Bu^t)-OBu^t insulin
IT : des-(B30) insulinyl-trypsin, acyl-enzyme

The concentrations of the Michaelis–Menten complexes of I, IA, IM, and IB with trypsin are denoted by I,T; IA,T; IM,T; and IB,T. The Michaelis–Menten complexes can react under formation of IT, viz. acyl-enzyme under release of water (k_{-W}), alanine (k_{-A}), Thr-OMe (k_{-M}), and Thr(Bu^t)-OBu^t (k_{-B}), respectively (see Figure 22).

Free trypsin, T, can associate with water, Thr-OMe or Thr(OBu^t)-OBu^t in the S$_1'$ site, under formation of T,W; T,M; and T,B; respectively. When the S$_1'$ site is occupied, insulin compounds having a B30 residue cannot associate under formation of Michaelis–Menten complexes. Des-(B30) insulin devoid of a B30 residue can bind with its Lys^{B29} residue to the S$_1$ site of trypsin independent of whatever ligand is bound to S$_1'$. Hence the strong inhibition Thr-OMe exerts on transpeptidation but not on coupling reactions is the result of a strong binding of Thr-OMe to the S$_1'$ subsite.

The acyl-enzyme IT, lacking the B30 residue, can bind water, Thr-OMe, and Thr(Bu^t)-OBu^t in its S$_1'$ site. Binding of the S$_1'$ ligands results in IT,W (K_W), IT,M (K_M) and IT,B (K_B) respectively. The release of alanine (k_{-A}) is considered irreversible, as the free alanine stabilizes in the zwitterion structure. Furthermore, it is available in a low concentration (8 mM) as compared to Thr-OMe and Thr(Bu^t)-OBu^t (1 M).

The seven first-order rate constants associated with the covalent reactions between the five complexes, IA,T, I,T, IM,T, IB,T and IT,W,M,B are denoted by k_{-A} (release of alanine), k_{-M} (release of Thr-OMe), k_M (uptake of Thr-OMe), k_{-B} (release of Thr(Bu^t)-OBu^t), k_B (uptake of Thr(Bu^t)-OBu^t, k_{-W} (release of water), and k_W (uptake of water).

Association and dissociation reactions are presumed to occur instantaneously, viz. fast compared to the covalent reactions. The quasi-equilibria are each described by an equilibrium dissociation constant:

(i) $$ IA + T \rightleftharpoons IA,T \qquad K_{IA} = \frac{IA \times T}{IA,T} $$

(ii) $$ IM + T \rightleftharpoons IM,T \qquad K_{IM} = \frac{IM \times T}{IM,T} $$

(iii)
$$IB + T \rightleftharpoons IB,T \qquad K_{IB} = \frac{IB \times T}{IB,T}$$

(iv)
$$I + T[0,W,M,B] \rightleftharpoons I,T[0,W,M,B]$$

$$K_I = \frac{I \times T[0,W,M,B]}{I,T[0,W,M,B]} = \frac{I \times T}{I,T}$$

As the insulins are present in a 40-fold excess relative to trypsin and since the K_m values are large, the concentrations of insulin compounds are, to a good approximation, equal to the total of the free and trypsin bound species IA $\simeq$ IA + IA,T, etc.

T [0,W,M,B] denotes T with free S_1' site or bound to water or Thr-OMe or Thr(Bu^t)-OBu^t, respectively.

As we have been unable to determine K_m constants because of the high degree of dissociation, the dissociation constants K_{IA}, K_{IM}, K_{IB}, and K_I have all been set at 0.1 M, which was the minimum estimate[71] for K_m. In this model, where associations and dissociations come to equilibrium instantaneously following covalent reactions, an increase in K_{IM} is equivalent to the proportional increase k_{-M}, etc. Hence, in the curve fitting procedures all insulin trypsin dissociation constants were kept at 0.1 M, while the k_{-A}, k_{-M}, k_{-B}, and k_{-W} were varied. The S_1' associations and dissociations between low molecular weight compounds and trypsin and insulinyl-trypsin are likewise in quasi-equilibria adapting to the covalent reactions and describable by equilibrium constants. It is furthermore presumed that the binding to the S_1' site has the same affinity in free trypsin and in insulinyl-trypsin:

(v)
$$T + W \rightleftharpoons T,W;$$

(vi)
$$IT + W \rightleftharpoons IT,W; \qquad K_W = \frac{T \times W}{T,W} = \frac{IT \times W}{IT,W}$$

(vii)
$$T + M \rightleftharpoons T,M;$$

(viii)
$$IT + M \rightleftharpoons IT,M; \qquad K_M = \frac{T \times M}{T,M} = \frac{IT \times M}{IT,M}$$

(ix)
$$T + B \rightleftharpoons T,B;$$

(x)
$$IT + B \rightleftharpoons IT,B; \qquad K_B = \frac{T \times B}{T,B} = \frac{IT \times B}{IT,B}$$

Having set the insulin-trypsin dissociation constants at 0.1 M, we are then left with the three equilibrium constants K_W, K_M, and K_B and the seven rate constants for fitting the model to simulate the reactions.

The fraction (μ) of free trypsin (T) is an algebraic function of W, M, B, I, IA, IM, IB, K_W, K_M, K_B, K_I, K_{IA}, K_{IM} and K_{IB}. Using (i, ii, iii, iv, vi, viii and x) this fraction $\mu = T/(T_0 - \Sigma IT)$, where T_0 denotes trypsin concentration at $t = 0$ and ΣIT the concentration of all species of insulinyl-trypsin, the equation derived is (xi):

(xi) $$\mu = \left[1 + \frac{W}{K_W} + \frac{M}{K_M} + \frac{B}{K_B} + \frac{I}{K_I} + \frac{IA}{K_{IA}} + \frac{IM}{K_{IM}} + \frac{IB}{K_{IB}}\right]^{-1}$$

The fractions of trypsin bound to IA, IM, IB and I, μ_{IA}, μ_{IM}, μ_{IB} and μ_I, respectively, are given by (xii, xiii, xiv and xv):

(xii) $$\mu_{IA} = \left[1 + \frac{K_{IA}}{IA}\left(1 + \frac{I}{K_I} + \frac{IM}{K_{IM}} + \frac{IB}{K_{IB}} + \frac{W}{K_W} + \frac{M}{K_M} + \frac{B}{K}\right)\right]^{-1}$$

(xiii) $$\mu_{IM} = \left[1 + \frac{K_{IM}}{IM}\left(1 + \frac{I}{K_I} + \frac{IA}{K_{IA}} + \frac{IB}{K_{IB}} + \frac{W}{K_W} + \frac{M}{K_M} + \frac{B}{K_B}\right)\right]^{-1}$$

(xiv) $$\mu_{IB} = \left[1 + \frac{K_{IB}}{IB}\left(1 + \frac{I}{K_I} + \frac{IA}{K_{IA}} + \frac{IM}{K_{IM}} + \frac{W}{K_W} + \frac{M}{K_M} + \frac{B}{K_B}\right)\right]^{-1}$$

(xv) $$\mu_I = \left[1 + \frac{K_I}{I}\left(1 + \frac{IA}{K_{IA}} + \frac{IM}{K_{IM}} + \frac{IB}{K_{IB}}\right)\right]^{-1}$$

The fraction of IT bound to M or B or W is likewise an algebraic function of the same constants. Using (vi, viii, and x) we derive (xvi, xvii, and xviii):

(xvi) $$\alpha_M = \frac{IT,M}{IT + IT,M + IT,B + IT,W}$$

$$= \frac{1}{1 + \dfrac{K_M}{M} + \dfrac{B \times K_M}{M \times K_B} + \dfrac{W \times K_M}{M \times K_W}}$$

(xvii) $$\alpha_B = \frac{IT,B}{IT + IT,B + IT,M + IT,W}$$

$$= \frac{1}{1 + \dfrac{K_B}{B} + \dfrac{M \times K_B}{B \times K_M} + \dfrac{W \times K_B}{B \times K_W}}$$

(xviii) $$\alpha_W = \frac{IT,W}{IT + IT,B + IT,M + IT,W}$$

$$= \frac{1}{1 + \dfrac{K_W}{W} + \dfrac{M \times K_W}{W \times K_M} + \dfrac{B \times K_W}{W \times K_B}}$$

Five rate equations correlate the covalent transformations between I, IA, IM, IB and IT, equation (xix) to (xxiii). The equations are:

(xix) $$\frac{dIA}{dt} = -k_{-A} \times IA,T = -k_{-A} \times \mu_{IA} \times (T_0 - \Sigma IT)$$

(xx) $\qquad \dfrac{dIM}{dt} = k_M \times IT,M - k_{-M} \times IM,T$

$\qquad = k_M \times \Sigma IT \times \alpha_M - k_{-M} \times \mu_{IM} \times (T_0 - \Sigma IT)$

(xxi) $\qquad \dfrac{dIB}{dt} = k_B \times IT,B - k_{-B} \times IB,T$

$\qquad = k_B \times \Sigma IT \times \alpha_B - k_{-B} \times \mu_{IB} \times (T_0 - \Sigma IT)$

(xxii) $\qquad \dfrac{dI}{dT} = k_W \times IT,W - k_{-W} \times I,T$

$\qquad = k_W \times \Sigma IT \times \alpha_W - k_{-W} \times \mu_I \times (T_0 - \Sigma IT)$

(xxiii) $\quad \dfrac{dIT}{dt} = (T_0 - \Sigma IT)[k_{-A} \times \mu_{IA} + k_{-M} \times \mu_{IM} + k_{-B} \times \mu_{IB} + k_{-W} \times \mu_I]$

$\qquad - \Sigma IT \times [k_M \times \alpha_M + k_B \times \alpha_B + k_W \times \alpha_W]$

Provided that W, M, B and T are constant during the reactions, the five rate equations can be solved as an eigenvalue problem using matrix mathematics. Since W, M and B are available in large excess relative to insulins and trypsin (11 M, 1 M and 1 M relative to 8 mM and 0.2 mM), W, M and B remain constant for all practical purposes. T will vary, especially at the beginning of a fast reaction where build-up of IT takes place. The eigenvalue problem is then solved at successive small time intervals, in which the concentration of T can be regarded as constant.

A program written in Pascal for IBM AT or TX personal computers was developed by B. Lautrup and M. Ålund, Scientific Consulting. The simulation of a reaction progress curve is a matter of a few minutes using this program, even though small steps in time must be taken at the beginning of a reaction where T is changing. For the fastest reaction encountered here, the coupling of I with M, 10 steps of 10^{-4} min followed by 10 steps of 10^{-3} min followed by 10 steps of 10^{-2} min and 100 steps of 0.2 min provided for a secure start with satisfactorily small changes of T, viz. less than 1% relatively within each segment. Thereafter intervals one or several minutes long can be taken without influencing the result of the simulation. This insensitivity of the step length is in contrast to our experience using numerical integration by the fourth-order Runge–Kutta methods, where small steps are essential throughout the simulation. Using the Kinsim program[121] on a VAX-11/780 we were able to simulate 3–4 hours' reaction progress using 10 minutes of CPU time. Using the APL program[71] on an IBM 4341 computer we were able to simulate 6 hours of reaction time using 8 hours of CPU time. Hence the efficiency in solving the rate equations rather than using numerical integration methods is obvious, especially when constants have to be fitted by trial and error. One cycle is completed in about 0.4 s using the IBM AT personal computer. The final equilibria between insulin compounds are defined by three sub-equilibria (xxiv–xxvi) and the mass conservation equation for insulin compounds (xxvii). Note that IA is zero at the final equilibrium. IX_0 denotes initial concentration of any insulin substrate.

(xxiv) $$k_W \times IT,W = k_{-W} \times I,T[0,W,M,B]$$

(xxv) $$k_M \times IT,M = k_{-M} \times IM,T$$

(xxvi) $$k_B \times IT,B = k_{-B} \times IB,T$$

(xxvii) $$IX_0 = [I + I,T] + [IM + IM,T] + [IB + IB,T] + \Sigma IT$$

Equations xxiv–xxvii are algebraic expressions of the rate and equilibrium constants. The product distribution of the four insulin compounds is calculated from the four equations by the Pascal program, independent of the reaction progress simulation. To control whether sufficiently small steps were taken during the initial phases of the progress simulation, a comparison can be made between the end result of the simulated progress curve and the solution of the four equilibrium equations (xxiv–xxvii) which give values for I, IM, IB and IT in equilibrium.

It was possible to simulate the reaction progress curves and to attain the correct equilibria in the experiments with only one threonine ester in the medium. One set of constants that resulted in simulation curves in good accordance with experimental data was:

Dissociation constants (M)	Rate constants (min^{-1})		$k_{cat}/K_{dissociation}$ (min^{-1}M^{-1})	
	k_2 Acylation	k_3 Deacylation	Acylation	Deacylation
$K_{insulins}$ = 0.1	k_{-A} = 39		390	
K_M = 0.04	k_{-M} = 301	k_M = 81	3010	2025
K_B = 0.172	k_{-B} = 26	k_B = 67	260	390
K_W = 11	k_{-W} = 192	k_W = 975	1920	89

The simulated curves for this set of constants of the various experiments plotted together with the experimental data are shown in Figures 28–33.

The comparisons between simulated curves and experimental data are shown for coupling reactions in Figures 28 and 29, and for transpeptidation reactions in Figures 30–32. Only the IB → IM reaction, Figure 33, fails to comply with the simulated reaction progress curve due to trypsin inactivation as discussed earlier. The calculated amounts of acyl-enzyme IT become 0.7% of the I in the I ⇌ IM equilibrium, and 0.2% of the I in the I ⇌ IB equilibrium. The accordance with the data is such that the model cannot be falsified from the data. The model closely simulates the coupling of I to IM (Figure 28) and the coupling of I to IB (Figure 29). The transpeptidation of IA to IM with nearly coinciding rises in IM and Ala is shown in Figure 30 and the transpeptidation of IA to IB, featuring a significant gap between IB and Ala, is shown in Figure 31. Transpeptidation of IM to IB results in an early peak of I, which eventually declines to equilibrium concentrations (Figure 32).

Simulations of the experiments with threonine esters in mixture in the reaction medium could not be brought into agreement with the experimental data, most markedly demonstrated in the state of equilibrium. The experiments consistently resulted in an IM/IB ratio of about 1.2 (Table 38, Figure 17), whereas the simulations, using constants that satisfy the equilibria in

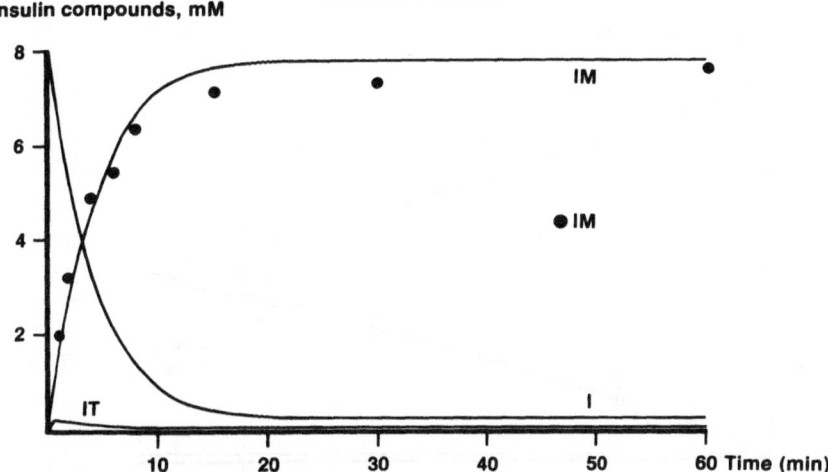

Figure 28 Simulation of reaction progress curve coupling DAI with Thr-OMe to yield HI-OMe, compared to experimental data. This is the fastest reaction encountered using the standard conditions. Simulated equilibrium: 2.7% I, 97.3% IM and 0.02% IT. The acyl-enzyme (IT) is depicted on an enlarged ordinate (10:1)

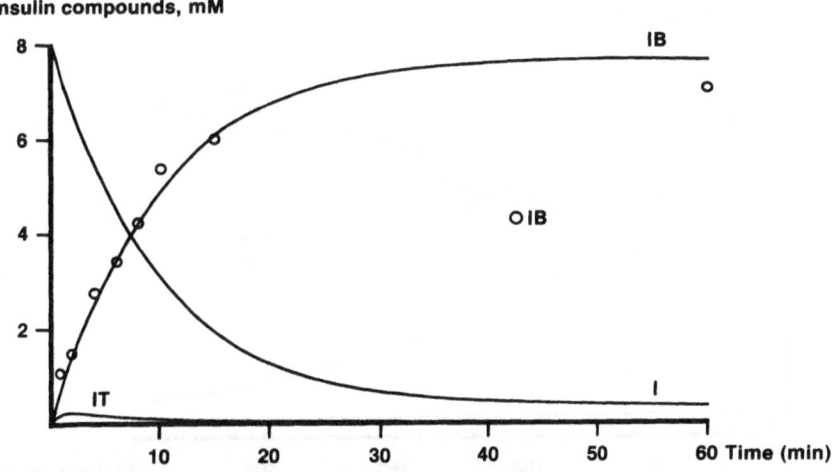

Figure 29 Simulation of reaction progress coupling DAI with Thr(Bu^t)-OBu^t to yield HI(Bu^t)-OBu^t, compared to experimental data. Simulated equilibrium 4.1% I, 95.9% IB and 0.01% IT. The acyl-enzyme (IT) is depicted on an enlarged ordinate (10:1)

experiments with separated threonine esters, result in an IM/IB ratio of about 0.44. The inadequacy of the model to simulate the experiments with mixed threonine esters is due to the implied, incorrect assumption of the two threonine esters reacting independently in the mixture. Since Thr(Bu^t)-OBu^t is a slightly stronger base than Thr-OMe (Table 1), the activity of Thr-OMe increases at the cost of the activity of Thr(Bu^t)-OBu^t as equilibrium (xxviii)

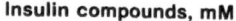
Insulin compounds, mM

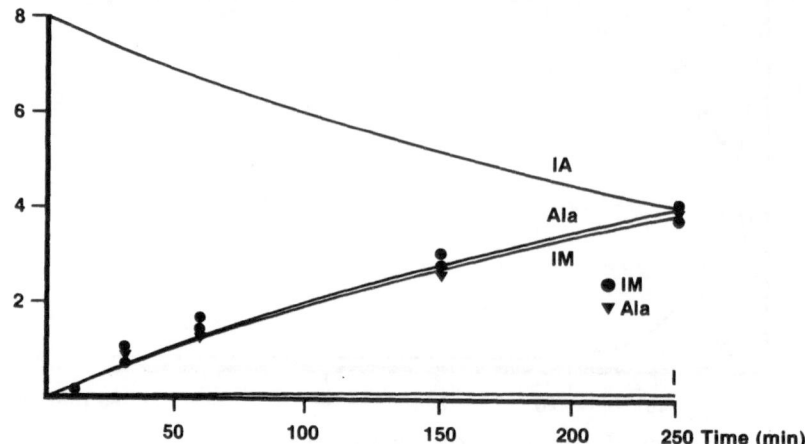

Figure 30 Simulation of reaction progress transpeptidizing porcine insulin to HI-OMe, compared to experimental data. Note the nearly coinciding values for Ala and HI-OMe. Simulated equilibrium: 2.7% I, 97.3% IM and 0.02% IT, cf. Figure 28.

Insulin compounds, mM

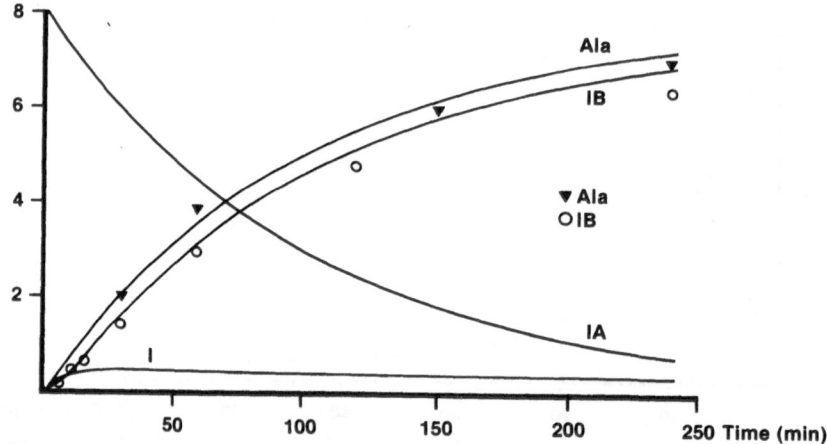

Figure 31 Simulation of reaction progress transpeptidizing porcine insulin to HI(Bu^t)-OBu^t, compared to experimental data. Note the noticeable gap between values for Ala and HI(Bu^t)-OBu^t and the transient peak in I. Simulated equilibrium: 4.1% I, 95.9% HB and 0.01% IT, cf. Figure 29

is displaced towards the right:

(xxviii) H^+-Thr-OMe + Thr(Bu^t)-OBu^t $\rightleftharpoons$ Thr-OMe + H^+-Thr(Bu^t)-OBu^t

Despite the inability of the model to cope with threonine esters interacting according to (xxviii), initial reaction progress is qualitatively simulated by

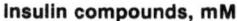

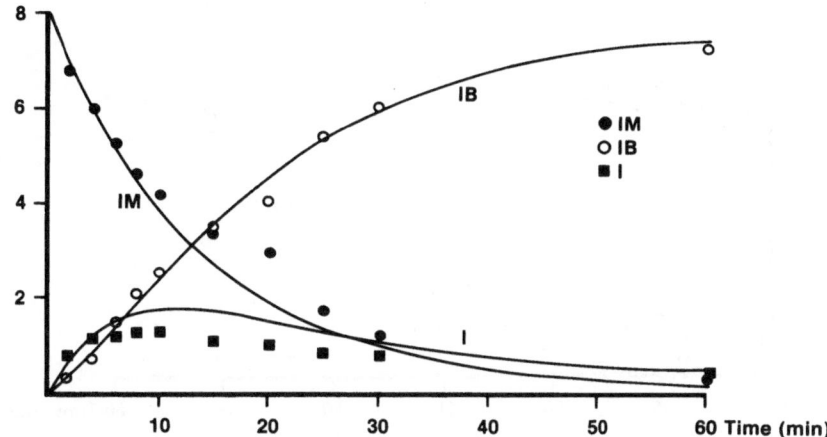

Figure 32 Simulation of reaction progress transpeptidizing HI-OMe to HI(Bu^t)-OBu^t, compared to experimental data. Note the transient maximum of DAI occurring at about 10 min. This is the fastest transpeptidation reaction encountered. Standard conditions. Simulated equilibrium: 4.1% I and 95.9% IB, same as in Figures 29 and 31

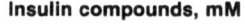

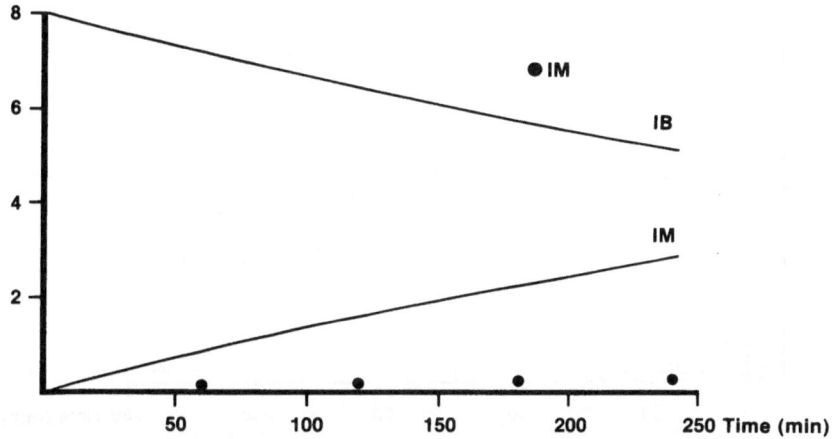

Figure 33 Simulation of the reaction progress transpeptidizing HI(Bu^t)-OBu^t to HI-OMe. This is the slowest transpeptidation reaction encountered using standard conditions. Due to trypsin inactivation, cf. Figure 27, the simulation cannot be fitted to comply with experimental data

the model using the above set of constants. The simulation of the coupling of I to yield a mixture of IM and IB shows the transient peak in IM (Figure 34).

The transpeptidation of IA to a mixture of IM and IB starts with a higher rate of formation of IM relative to IB, as observed experimentally (Figure

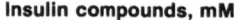

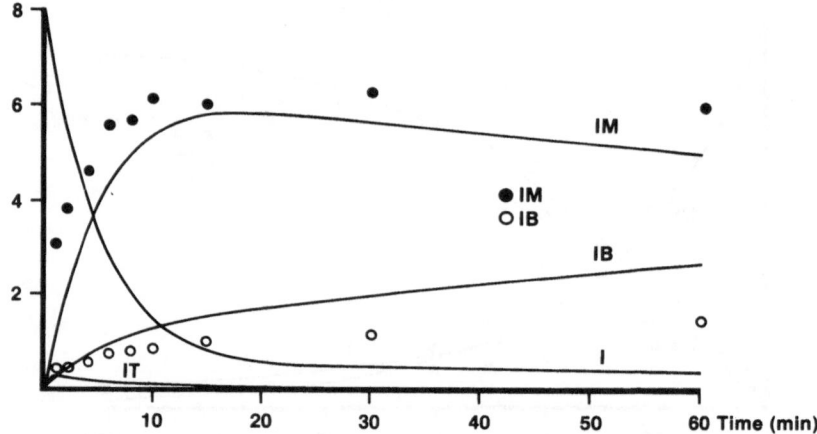

Figure 34 Simulation of reaction progress coupling DAI with a mixture of Thr-OMe and Thr(Bu^t)-OBu^t, yielding HI-OMe and HI(Bu^t)-OBu^t, compared to experimental data. Note the transient maximum of HI-OMe. Actual equilibrium: 3.3% I, 53.4% IM and 43.3% IB. Simulated equilibrium: 2.6% I, 29.8% IM, 67.6% IB and 0.01% IT. The acyl-enzyme (IT) is depicted on an enlarged ordinate (10:1)

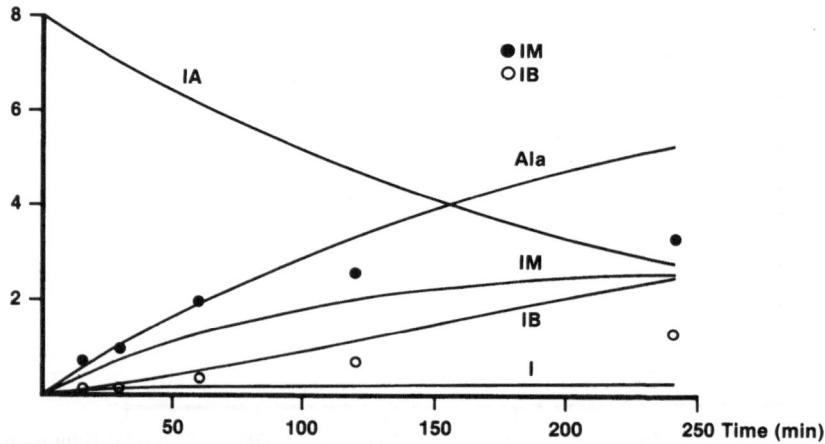

Figure 35 Simulation of reaction progress transpeptidizing porcine insulin to mixtures of HI-OMe and HI(Bu^t)-OBu^t, compared to experimental data. Note the slow initial increase in HI(Bu^t)-OBu^t. Actual equilibrium: 3.3% I, 53,4% IM and 43.3% IB. Simulated equilibrium: 2.6% I, 29.8% IM, 67.6% IB and 0.01% IT

35). The initial rate ratio of 10 observed experimentally (Figure 23) is reduced to about 5 in the simulation, due to the lack of incorporation of threonine ester interaction in the model.

If the activities of Thr-OMe and Thr(Bu^t)-OBu^t in the mixed experiments are put at 0.73 M and 0.27 M, respectively, an equilibrium ratio of 1.19

Insulin compounds, mM

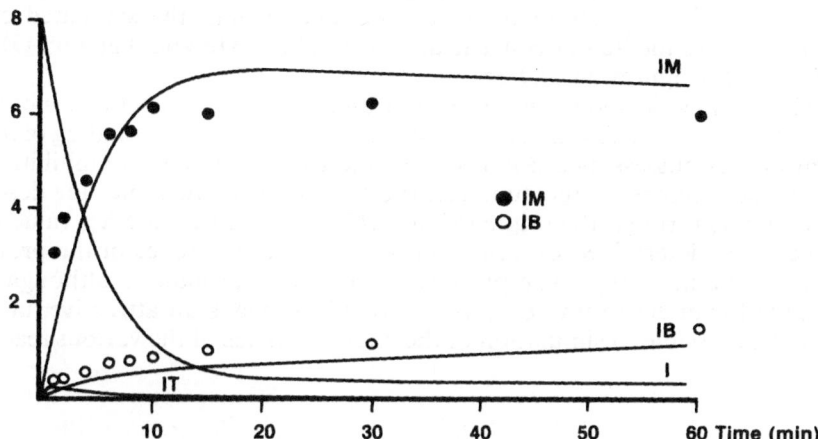

Figure 36 Simulated reaction progress curves of the I to IM + IB coupling reaction, using activities for Thr-OMe and Thr(Bu^t)-OBu^t of 0.73 M and 0.27 M in the simulation, whereas the actual concentrations were 0.5 M for both threonine esters. The corresponding simulation, using the actual concentrations, is shown in Figure 34. Actual equilibrium: 3.3% I, 53.4% IM and 43.3% IB. Simulated equilibrium: 2.5% I, 53.0% IM, 44.5% IB and 0.02% IT. The acyl-enzyme (IT) is depicted on an enlarged ordinate (10:1)

Insulin compounds, mM

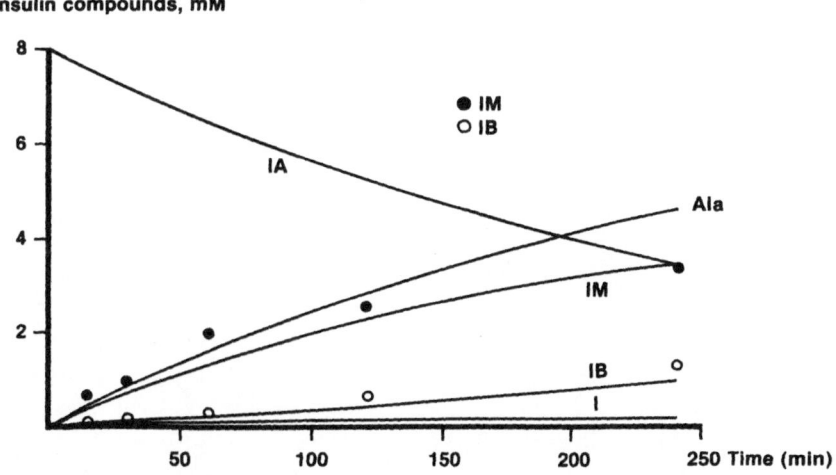

Figure 37 Simulated reaction progress curves for the IA to IM + IB transpeptidation reaction, using activities for Thr-OMe and Thr(Bu^t)-OBu^t of 0.73 M and 0.27 M in the simulation, whereas the actual concentrations were 0.5 M for both threonine esters. The corresponding simulation, using the actual concentrations, is shown in Figure 35. Actual equilibrium: 3.3% I, 53.4% IM and 43.3% IB. Simulated equilibrium: 2.5% I, 53.0% IM, 44.5% IB and 0.02% IT.

95

between IM and IB is derived using the same set of constants. The simulated reaction progress curves for coupling (Figure 36) and for transpeptidation (Figure 37) fit the experimental data far better than the simulated curves derived using the actual concentrations of Thr-OMe and Thr(Bu^t)-OBu^t of 0.5 M each (Figures 34 and 35).

The proposed model comprises a straightforward competitive inhibition, where the second substrate, the threonine ester, inhibits the binding of insulin compounds possessing a B30 residue. Due to this competitive inhibition the K_m values increase. Unfortunately, the Lineweaver–Burk plot for des-(B30) insulin cuts through the origin (Figure 26), meaning that the K_m value is too large to be determined experimentally even in the absence of the proposed competitive inhibition. The proposed inhibition mechanism, although inaccessible for direct testing by classical plots, provides an attractive, unifying model, accessible to simulation of the characteristics of the various reactions.

7
Summary

Threonine^{B30} esters of human insulin are made from porcine insulin and biosynthetic, single-chain precursors in satisfactory yields making production of human insulin possible on the basis of each type of substance. The substances are transpeptidized by means of trypsin in a mixture of water and an organic solvent with a threonine ester, e.g.:

(i) Porcine insulin + Thr-OR $\xrightarrow{\text{trypsin}}$ Thr^{B30}-OR human insulin + Ala

(ii) B(1–29)-A(1–21) insulin + Thr-OR $\xrightarrow{\text{trypsin}}$ Thr^{B30}-OR human insulin

Specificity for the desired reaction is induced because the penultimate residue of the B-chain, B29, is lysine. However, the specificity is not absolute, as residue B22 is arginine. This means that hydrolysis and transpeptidation at B22 lead to loss of insulin in the form of desoctapeptide-(B23-B30) insulin and its threonine ester.

Additional circumstances cause the yield of human insulin ester to be less than 100% in practice. Even though a large molar excess of threonine ester compared to insulin is used, and even though the activity of water is reduced by adding organic solvents, it is not possible to displace the equilibrium (iii) totally to the right:

(iii)   Des-(B30) insulin + Thr-OR $\underset{\text{trypsin}}{\rightleftharpoons}$ Thr^{B30}-OR insulin + H$_2$O

The activity of trypsin is greatly reduced in the aqueous–organic medium, and an irreversible autolysis occurs. Consequently, the transpeptidation reactions become slow, and chemical by-product formation, e.g. deamidation of Asn^{A21} and ester hydrolysis of Thr^{B30}-OMe insulin, further reduces yields during the long reaction time.

The specificity defined as $k(\text{Lys}^{B29})/k(\text{Arg}^{B22})$ is found to increase (a) with a reduced concentration of water in the medium, (b) with an increased concentration of a weak organic acid in the reaction mixture, (c) with a reduced temperature, and (d) when using strongly polar solvents like DMF and DMAC instead of alcohols. Transpeptidation reactions with good yields have been conducted at temperatures as low as $-20°$C.

The equilibrium (iii) can be displaced to more than 97% synthesis of Thr^{B30}-OR insulin, e.g. by using 20% H$_2$O, 1 M threonine ester, and DMAC as solvents. The strongly polar, aprotic solvents displace the equilibrium (iii) more effectively to the right than, for example alcohols, acetone and THF with the same concentration of water. This means that the activity of water is being more reduced and/or the pK of the carboxylic acid group of Lys^{B29} more increased in DMF and DMAC than in alcohols.

The stability of trypsin in an organic–aqueous medium is increased by addition of Ca^{2+} as in aqueous solution. Addition of acid increases the stability, but causes reversible inactivation similar to that known from aqueous trypsin solutions. Of decisive importance for good yields is the use of temperatures considerably below the usual 25 or 37°C, as the autolysis of the trypsin is far more dependent on temperature than the rate of transpeptidation. When temperatures below 25°C are used the stability increases with the concentration of water in the range of 20–30%.

Considering the specificity, the position of the equilibrium, the stability of the trypsin, and the rate of the reaction, the selection of the optimal reaction conditions becomes a compromise. When porcine insulin is transpeptidized (i), the reaction rate is high enough for the specificity problem to be solved by using a large excess of acetic acid compared to threonine ester, e.g. 2.5 to 1 (M/M).

A single-chain insulin derivative, B(1–29)-A(1–21), was made by trans-peptidizing porcine insulin in the absence of threonine esters. It was shown *in vitro* that the disulphide bridges in this single-chain insulin precursor could be reduced and reoxidized, regenerating the substance in better yields than when using porcine proinsulin. This ability is also found *in vivo*, as the compound can be expressed in yeast by recombinant DNA techniques.

The reaction rate is reduced considerably in the transpeptidation of single-chain insulins to human insulin esters. The short bridge between the A- and the B-chains in the biosynthetic, single-chain insulin precursors induces a steric hindrance for the transpeptidation reaction (ii). The specificity is a bigger problem than when transpeptidizing porcine insulin, as the two cleavable bonds, Arg^{B22}-Gly^{B23} and Lys^{B29}-Gly^{A1}, become very similar with regard to k values. The problem of the slow transpeptidation of the Lys^{B29}-Gly^{A1} linkage can be solved by using equimolar amounts of Thr-OMe and acetic acid besides inserting a few additional amino acids between the chains. Two such biosynthetic precursors, which can be transpeptidized to human insulin ester more easily than B(1–29)-A(1–21) insulin, are B(1–29)-Ala-Ala-Lys-A(1–21) insulin and B(1–29)-Ser-Lys-A(1–21) insulin. Porcine proinsulin, which has 34 amino acids between Lys^{B29} and Gly^{A1}, can be transpeptidized at least as fast as porcine insulin.

It is also possible to speed up the slow transpeptidation of B(1–29)-A(1–21) insulin to a human insulin ester by using Thr(Bu^t)-OBu^t instead of Thr-OMe. By using 1 M Thr(Bu^t)-OBu^t and 2.5 M acetic acid, a reasonably fast and reasonably specific reaction can be carried out with a yield of 90%. The use of equimolar amounts of Thr(Bu^t)-OBu^t and acetic acid leads to heavy formation of desoctapeptide in contrast to the use of equimolar amounts of Thr-OMe and acetic acid. The marked difference between the two threonine esters is also seen when the k values for transpeptidation and coupling, reactions (i) and (iii), are compared. Transpeptidation proceeds faster with Thr(Bu^t)-OBu^t than with Thr-OMe, whereas the opposite is the case in coupling. In reactions using a mixture of equimolar amounts of Thr-OMe and Thr(Bu^t)-OBu^t, Thr^{B30}-OMe human insulin initially increases faster than Thr^{B30}(Bu^t)-OBu^t human insulin in coupling as well as in transpeptidation reactions, while a ratio between the two human insulin esters of about 1.2 is established in the equilibrium. A model has been set up that qualitatively and quantitatively simulates the coupling and transpeptidation reactions between des-(B30) insulin, porcine insulin, Thr^{B30}-OMe insulin, and Thr^{B30}(Bu^t)-OBu^t insulin. The inhibitory effect of Thr-OMe on transpeptidation, but not on coupling reactions, is dealt with as a competitive binding of Thr-OMe to the subsite S_1' of the trypsin, excluding binding of insulins with an amino acid in position B30, whereas des-(B30) insulin is still able to bind independent of S_1' occupancy. Threonine esters and water compete in binding to the S_1' site of the acyl-enzyme, des-(B30) insulinyl-trypsin. According to the model Thr-OMe binds better than Thr(Bu^t)-OBu^t to S_1'. It is thus explained how Thr-OMe inhibits trans-peptidation to a higher extent than Thr(Bu^t)-OBu^t, as well as how Thr-OMe couples faster than Thr(Bu^t)-OBu^t. The reactions using threonine esters in mixture require a correction for proton exchange between the threonine esters in order to fit the model quantitatively.

The activity of trypsin in organic–aqueous solutions is strongly reduced in relation to its activity in aqueous solutions. In accordance with this, large K_m values (> 0.1 M) are found, meaning that the reduced activity can at least partly be accounted for by a large dissociation constant in the equilibrium, (iv):

(iv)
$$\text{Insulin} + \text{trypsin} \overset{\text{trypsin}}{\rightleftharpoons} \text{insulin, trypsin}$$

K_m values were too large to be determined experimentally.

8
Resumé

Threonin^{B30} estere af humaninsulin er fremstillet ud fra svineinsulin og ud fra biosyntetiske, enkeltkædede forstadier i så gode udbytter, at produktion af humaninsulin er blevet mulig ud fra begge typer af udgangsstoffer. Udgangsstofferne transpeptideres ved hjælp af trypsin i en blanding af vand og et organisk opløsningsmiddel med en threoninester f.eks.:

(i)   Svineinsulin + Thr-OR $\xrightarrow{\text{trypsin}}$ Thr^{B30}-OR humaninsulin + Ala

(ii)   B(1–29)-A(1–21) insulin + Thr-OR $\xrightarrow{\text{trypsin}}$ Thr^{B30}-OR humaninsulin

Specificiteten i reaktionen fremkommer ved, at den næstsidste aminosyre i B-kæden, B29, er lysin. Specificiteten er dog ikke absolut, idet aminosyre B22 er arginin, således at såvel hydrolyse som transpeptidering ved B22 fører til tab af insulin i form af desoktapeptid-(B23-B30) insulin og dets threoninester.

Der er yderligere en række årsager til, at udbyttet af human insulinester i praksis bliver mindre end 100%. Selv om der anvendes stort molært overskud af threoninester i forhold til insulin, og selv om aktiviteten af vand reduceres ved tilsætning of organiske opløsningsmidler, kan ligevægten (iii) ikke forskydes totalt til højre:

(iii)   Des-(B30) insulin + Thr-OR $\xrightleftharpoons{\text{trypsin}}$ Thr^{B30}-OR insulin + H$_2$O

Trypsin har stærkt nedsat aktivitet i vandige organiske blandinger og autolyserer desuden irreversibelt. Følgelig bliver transpeptideringsreaktionerne langsomme, og kemiske bireaktioner såsom deamidering af Asn^{A21} og esterhydrolyse af Thr^{B30}-OMe insulin vil sideløbende formindske udbytterne.

Specificiteten defineret som $k(\text{Lys}^{B29})/k(\text{Arg}^{B22})$ findes at stige (a) med nedsat koncentration af vand i blandinger, (b) med forøget koncentration af en svag organisk syre i reaktionsblandingen, (c) med nedsat temperatur, og (d) ved anvendelse af stœrkt polære opløsningsmidler som DMF og DMAC fremfor alkoholer. Der er gennemført transpeptideringsreaktioner i godt udbytte ved temperaturer ned til − 20°C.

Ligevægten (iii) kan forskydes til mere end 97% syntese af Thr^{B30}-OR insulin, f.eks. ved anvendelse af 20% H$_2$O, 1 M threoninester og DMAC som opløsningsmiddel. Stærkt polære, aprotiske opløsningsmidler forskyder ligevægten (iii) mere effektivt til højre end f.eks. alkoholer, acetone og THF for samme koncentration af vand, d.v.s. at aktiviteten af vand reduceres mere og/eller pK af carboxylgruppen af Lys^{B29} forøges mere i DMF og DMAC end i alkoholer.

Stabiliteten af trypsin i organisk-vandigt medium forøges ved tilsætning af Ca^{2+} som i vandig opløsning. Tilsætning af syre forøger stabiliteten, men forårsager reversibel inaktivering i lighed med hvad der er kendt fra vandige trypsinopløsninger. Afgørende for gode udbytter er anvendelse af temperaturer væsentligt under de sædvanligvis anvendte 25 eller 37°C, idet trypsinets autolyse er langt mere temperaturafhængig end k reaktionshastigheden af transpeptidering. Ved temperaturer under 25°C stiger stabiliteten med koncentrationen af vand i området mellem 20 og 30%.

Fastlæggelse af optimale reaktionsbetingelser under hensyntagen til specificitet, ligevægtens beliggenhed, trypsinets stabilitet samt reaktionens hastighed bliver således et kompromis. Ved transpeptidering af svineinsulin (i), er reaktionshastigheden så rimelig stor, at specificitetsproblemet kan løses ved at anvende stort overskud af eddikesyre i forhold til threoninester f.eks. 2.5 til 1 (M/M).

Et enkeltkædet insulinderivat, B(1–29)-A(1–21), blev fremstillet ved transpeptidering af svineinsulin i fravær af threoninestre. Det blev demonstreret *in vitro*, at svovlbroerne i dette enkeltkædede insulinforstadie kunne reduceres og reoxyderes under gendannelse af stoffet i bedre udbytte end svineproinsulin. Denne egenskab genfindes *in vivo*, idet stoffet kan udtrykkes i gær ved hjælp af rekombinant DNA teknik.

Ved transpeptidering af de biosyntetiske, enkeltkædede insulinforstadier (ii) giver den korte bro mellem A- og B-kæden en sterisk hindring, således at reaktionshastigheden reduceres betydeligt. Specificiteten bliver et større problem end ved transpeptidering af svineinsulin, idet de 2 spaltningssteder Arg^{B22}-Gly^{B23} og Lys^{B29}-Gly^{A1} bliver meget ens m.h.t. k værdier. Problemet med den langsomme transpeptidering ved Lys^{B29}-Gly^{A1} bindingen kan løses ved at anvende ved ækvimolære mængder af Thr-OMe og eddikesyre samt ved at indskyde et par ekstra aminosyrer mellem kæderne. To sådanne biosyntetiske forstadier, som hurtigere kan transpeptideres til humaninsulinester end B(1–29)-A(1–21) insulin, er B(1–29)-Ala-Ala-Lys-A(1–21) insulin og B(1–29)-Ser-Lys-A(1–21) insulin. Svineproinsulin, som har 34 aminosyrer mellem Lys^{B29} og Gly^{A1}, transpeptideres lige så hurdigt som svineinsulin.

En anden måde at fremskynde den langsomme transpeptidering af B(1–29)-A(1–21) insulin til en human insulinester er at anvende $Thr(Bu^t)$-OBu^t med stedet for Thr-OMe. Ved anvendelse af 1 M $Thr(Bu^t)$-OBu^t og 2.5 M eddikesyre kan en rimelig hurtig og rimelig specifik reaktion gennemføres med 90% udbytte. Anvendelse af ækvimolære mængder af $Thr(Bu^t)$-OBu^t og eddikesyre fører til kraftig desoktapeptiddannelse i modsætning til anvendelse af ækvimolære mængder af Thr-OMe og eddikesyre. Den markante forskel mellem de to threoninestre ses også ved en sammenligning af k værdier for transpeptidering og kobling, reaktionerne (i) og (iii). Transpeptidering forløber hurtigere med $Thr(Bu^t)$-OBu^t end med Thr-OMe, medens det omvendte er tilfældet ved kobling. I forsøg med ækvimolære mængder Thr-OMe og Thr(Bu^t)-OBu^t i blanding syntetiseres Thr^{B30}-OMe humaninsulin hurtigere end Thr^{B30}(Bu^t)-OBu^t humaninsulin i begyndelsen i såvel koblings- som transpeptideringsreaktioner, medens ligevægten etableres med et forhold på omkring 1,2 mellem de to humaninsulinestere. Der opstilles en model som kvalitativt og kvantitativt simulerer koblings- og transpeptideringsreaktionerne mellem des-(B30) insulin, svineinsulin, Thr^{B30}-OMe insulin og Thr^{B30}(Bu^t)-OBu^t insulin. Den inhiberende virkning af Thr-OMe på transpeptidering, men ikke på koblingsreaktioner, fortolkes som en kompetitiv binding af Thr-OMe til trypsinets subsite S$_1'$, hvorved binding af insuliner, som har en aminosyre i position B30, udelukkes, hvorimod des-(B30) insulin stadigvæk kan bindes. I acyl-enzymet, des-(B30) insulinyl-trypsin, er binding af threoninestre mulig. Da Thr-OMe ifølge modellen bindes bedre end Thr(Bu^t)-OBu^t til S$_1'$, forklares såvel at Thr-OMe hæmmer transpeptidering, som at Thr-OMe kobler hurtigere. I forsøgene med threoninestere i blanding kræves en korrektion for protonudveksling mellem disse for at tilpasse forsøgene kvantitativt til modellen.

Trypsinets aktivitet i de organisk-vandige opløsninger er stærkt reduceret i forhold til dets aktivitet i vandig opløsning. I overensstemmelse hermed findes store K_m værdier (>0.1 M), således at den nedsatte aktivitet i hvert fald delvist kan forklares med en stor dissociationskonstant i ligevægten (iv):

(iv) $$\text{Insulin} + \text{trypsin} \overset{\text{trypsin}}{\rightleftharpoons} \text{insulin, trypsin}$$

K_m værdier var for store til at kunne bestemmes eksperimentelt.

References

1. Markussen, J. (1984). Production of human insulin. In Nattrass, M. and Santiago, J. V. (eds.) *Recent Advances in Diabetes*, **1**, 45–53
2. Chance, R. E., Hoffmann, J. A., Kroeff, E. P., Johnson, M. G., Schirmer, E. W. and Bromer, W. W. (1981). The production of human insulin using recombinant DNA technology and a new chain combination procedure. In Rich, D. H. and Gross, E. (eds.) *Peptides. Synthesis – Structure – Function.* Proceedings of the *seventh American Peptide Symposium.* pp. 721–8. Rockford, Ill.: Pierce Chemical Company.
3. Heding, L. G., Marshall, M. O., Persson, B., Dahlquist, G., Thalme, B., Lindgren, F., Åkerblom, H. K., Rilva, A., Knip, M., Ludvigsson, J., Stenhammar, L., Strömberg, L., Søvik, O., Bævre, H., Wefring, K., Vidnes, J., Kjærgård, J. J., Bro, P. and Kaad, P. H. (1984). Immunogenicity of monocomponent human and porcine insulin in newly diagnosed type 1 (insulin-dependent) diabetic children. *Diabetologia*, **27**, 96–8
4. Falholt, K., Hoskam, J. A. M., Karamanos, B. G., Süsstrunk, H., Viswanathan, M. and Heding, L. G. (1983). Insulin-specific IgE in serum of 67 diabetic patients against human insulin (Novo), porcine insulin, and bovine insulin. Four case reports. *Diabetes Care*, **6** suppl. 1, 61–5
5. Borsook, H. (1953). Peptide bond formation. In Anson, M. L., Bailey, K. and Edsall, J. T. (eds.) *Adv. Protein Chem.* **8**, 127–74
6. Carpenter, F. H. (1960). The free energy change in hydrolytic reactions: the non-ionized compound convention. *J. Am. Chem. Soc.* **82**, 1111–22
7. Huffman, H. M. (1941). Thermal data. XIV. The heat capacities and entropies of some compounds having the peptide bond. *J. Am. Chem. Soc.*, **63**, 688–9
8. Huffman, H. M. (1942). Thermal data. XV. The heats of combustion and free energies of some compounds containing the peptide bond. *J. Phys. Chem.*, **46**, 885–91
9. Linderstrøm-Lang, K. (1951). Lane Medical Lectures. V. Biological synthesis of proteins. In *Selected Papers.* pp. 448–71. (New York, London (1962): Academic Press)
10. Dobry, A., Fruton, J. S. and Sturtevant, J. M. (1952). Thermodynamics of hydrolysis of peptide bonds. *J. Biol. Chem.*, **195**, 149–54
11. Michaelis, L. and Mizutani, M. (1925). Die Dissociation der schwachen Elektrolyte in wässerig-alkoholischen Lösungen. *Z. Phys. Chem.*, **116**, 135–59
12. Mizutani, M. (1925). Die Dissociation der schwachen Elektrolyte in wässerig-alkoholischen Lösungen. II. Die Beziehungen zwischen chemischer Konstitution und Alkoholempfindlichkeit der Saüren und Basen. *Z. Phys. Chem.*, **116**, 350–8
13. Butler, L. G. and Reithel, F. J. (1977) Urease-catalyzed urea synthesis. *Arch. Biochem. Biophys.*, **178**, 43–50
14. Homandberg, G. A., Mattis, J. A. and Laskowski, M. (1978). Synthesis of peptide bonds by proteinases. Addition of organic cosolvents shifts peptide bond equilibria toward synthesis. *Biochemistry*, **17**, 5220–7
15. Sealock, R. W. and Laskowski, M. (1969). Enzymatic replacement of the arginyl by a lysyl residue in the reactive site of soybean trypsin inhibitor. *Biochemistry*, **8**, 3703–10
16. Kowalski, D., Leary, T. R., McKee, R. E., Sealock, R. W., Wang, D. and Laskowski, M. (1974). Replacements, insertions, and modifications of amino acid residues in the reactive site of soybean trypsin inhibitor (Kunitz). In Fritz, H., Tschesche, H., Greene, L. J. and Truscheit, E. (eds.) *Proteinase Inhibitors.* Proceedings of the *2nd International Research Conference, Bayer-Symposium V.* pp. 311–24. (Berlin, Heidelberg, New York: Springer-Verlag)

17. Bender, M. L., Clement, G. E., Gunter, C. R. and Kézdy, F. J. (1964). The kinetics of α-chymotrypsin reactions in the presence of added nucleophiles. *J. Am. Chem. Soc.*, **86**, 3697–703

18. Fink, A. L. and Bender, M. L. (1969). Binding sites for substrate leaving groups and added nucleophiles in papain-catalyzed hydrolyses. *Biochemistry*, **8**, 5109–18

19. Breddam, K. and Ottesen, M. (1984). Malt carboxypeptidase catalyzed ammonolysis reactions. *Carlsberg Res. Commun.*, **49**, 473–81

20. Riechmann, L. and Kasche, V. (1985). Peptide synthesis catalyzed by serine proteinases chymotrypsin and trypsin. *Biochim. Biophys. Acta*, **830**, 164–72

21. Fastrez, J. and Fersht, A. R. (1973). Demonstration of the acyl-enzyme mechanism for the hydrolysis of peptides and anilides by chymotrypsin. *Biochemistry*, **12**, 2025–34

22. Blow, D. M. (1976). Structure and mechanism of chymotrypsin. *Accounts Chem. Res.*, **9**, 145–52

23. Wasteneys, H. and Borsook, H. (1930). The enzymatic synthesis of protein. *Physiol. Rev.*, **10**, 110–45

24. Bergmann, M. and Fraenkel-Conrat, H. (1937). The role of specificity in the enzymatic synthesis of proteins. *J. Biol. Chem.*, **119**, 707–20

25. Bergmann, M. and Fruton, J. S. (1938). Some synthetic and hydrolytic experiments with chymotrypsin. *J. Biol. Chem.*, **124**, 321–9

26. Bergmann, M. and Fraenkel-Conrat, H. (1938). The enzymatic synthesis of peptide bonds. *J. Biol. Chem.*, **124**, 1–6

27. Borsook, H. and Dubnoff, J. W. (1940). The biological synthesis of hippuric acid in vitro. *J. Biol. Chem.*, **132**, 307–24

28. Lipmann, F. (1941). Metabolic generation and utilization of phosphate bond energy. *Adv. Enzymol.*, **1**, 99–162

29. Bergmann, M. and Fruton, J. S. (1944). The significance of coupled reactions for the enzymatic hydrolysis and synthesis of proteins. *Ann. NY Acad. Sci.*, **45**, 409–23

30. Borsook, H. and Deasy, C. L. (1951). The metabolism of proteins and amino acids. *Annu. Rev. Biochem.*, **20**, 209–26

31. Fruton, J. S. (1950). The role of proteolytic enzymes in the biosynthesis of peptide bonds. *Yale J. Biol. Med.*, **22**, 263–71

32. Johnston, R. B., Mycek, M. J. and Fruton, J. S. (1950). Catalysis of transamidation reactions by proteolytic enzymes. *J. Biol. Chem.*, **185**, 629–41

33. Johnston, R. B., Mycek, M. J. and Fruton, J. S. (1950). Catalysis of transpeptidation reactions by chymotrypsin. *J. Biol. Chem.*, **187**, 205–11

34. Fruton, J. S., Johnston, R. B. and Fried, M. (1951). Elongation of peptide chains in enzyme-catalyzed transamidation reactions. *J. Biol. Chem.*, **190**, 39–53

35. Brenner, M., Müller, H. R. and Pfister, R. W. (1950). Eine neue enzymatische Peptidsynthese. *Helv. Chim. Acta*, **33**, 568–91

36. Widmer, F. and Johansen, J. T. (1979). Enzymatic peptide synthesis. Carboxypeptidase Y catalyzed formation of peptide bonds. *Carlsberg Res. Commun.*, **44**, 37–46

37. Breddam, K., Widmer, F. and Johansen, J. T. (1980). Carboxypeptidase Y catalyzed transpeptidations and enzymatic peptide synthesis. *Carlsberg Res. Commun.*, **45**, 237–47

38. Widmer, F., Breddam, K. and Johansen, J. T. (1980). Carboxypeptidase Y catalyzed peptide synthesis using amino acid alkyl esters as amine components. *Carlsberg Res. Commun.*, **45**, 453–63

39. Widmer, F., Breddam, K. and Johansen, J. T. (1981). Influence of the structure of amine components on carboxypeptidase Y catalyzed amide bond formation. *Carlsberg Res. Commun.*, **46**, 97–106

40. Breddam, K. (1986). Serine carboxypeptidases. A review. *Carlsberg Res. Commun.*, **51**, 83–128

41. Oka, T. and Morihara, K. (1977). Trypsin as a catalyst for peptide synthesis. *J. Biochem.*, **82**, 1055–62

42. Oka, T. and Morihara, K. (1978). Peptide bond synthesis catalyzed by α-chymotrypsin. *J. Biochem.*, **84**, 1277–83

43. Oka, T. and Morihara, K. (1980). Peptide bond synthesis catalyzed by thermolysin. *J. Biochem.* **88**, 807–13

44. Morihara, K. and Oka, T. (1981). Peptide bond synthesis catalyzed by subtilisin, papain, and pepsin. *J. Biochem.*, **89**, 385–95

REFERENCES

45. Ingalls, R. G., Squires, R. G. and Butler, L. G. (1975). Reversal of enzymatic hydrolysis: rate and extent of ester synthesis as catalyzed by chymotrypsin and subtilisin Carlsberg at low water concentrations. *Biotechnol. Bioeng.*, **17**, 1627–37

46. Laskowski, M. (1978). The use of proteolytic enzymes for the synthesis of specific peptide bonds in globular proteins. In Offord, R. E. and Di Bello, C. (eds.) *Semisynthetic Peptides and Proteins.* pp. 255–62. (London, New York, San Francisco: Academic Press)

47. Chaiken, I. M., Komoriya, A., Ohno, M. and Widmer, F. (1982). Use of enzymes in peptide synthesis. *Appl. Biochem. Biotechnol.* **7**, 385–99

48. Fruton, J. S. (1982). Proteinase-catalyzed synthesis of peptide bonds. *Adv. Enzymol.*, **53**, 239–306

49. Jakubke, H.-D., Kuhl, P. and Könnecke, A. (1985). Basic principles of protease-catalyzed peptide bond formation. *Angew. Chem. Int. Ed. Engl.*, **24**, 85–93

50. Nicol, D. S. H. W. and Smith, L. F. (1960). Amino-acid sequence of human insulin. *Nature*, **187**, 483–5

51. Brown, H., Sanger, F. and Kitai, R. (1955). The structure of pig and sheep insulins. *Biochem. J.*, **60**, 556–65

52. Ruttenberg, M. A. (1972). Human insulin: facile synthesis by modification of porcine insulin. *Science*, **177**, 623–6

53. König, W. and Volk, A. (1977). Succinimidbildung bei der Synthese des Insulin-A-Ketten(14-21)-Octapeptids. *Chem. Ber.*, **110**, 1–11

54. Obermeier, R. and Geiger, R. (1976). A new semisynthesis of human insulin. *Hoppe-Seyler's Z. Physiol. Chem.*, **357**, 759–67

55. Bodanszky, M. and Fried, J. (1966). US patent 3,276,961

56. Inouye, K., Watanabe, K., Morihara, K., Tochino, Y., Kanaya, T., Emura, J. and Sakakibara, S. (1979). Enzyme-assisted semisynthesis of human insulin. *J. Am. Chem. Soc.*, **101**, 751–2

57. Schmitt, E. W. and Gattner, H.-G. (1978). Verbesserte Darstellung von Des-alanyl^{B30}-insulin. *Hoppe-Seyler's Z. Physiol. Chem.*, **359**, 799–802

58. Slobin, L. I. and Carpenter, F. H. (1963). Action of carboxypeptidase-A on bovine insulin: preparation of desalanine-desasparagine-insulin. *Biochemistry*, **2**, 16–28

59. Morihara, K., Oka, T., Tsuzuki, H., Inouye, K. and Sakakibara, S. (1979). Semisynthesis of human insulin: trypsin-catalyzed replacement of alanine B30 by threonine in porcine insulin. In Gross, E. (ed.) Proceedings of the sixth American Peptide Symposium. pp. 617–20. (Rockford, Ill.: Pierce Chemical Company)

60. Morihara, K., Oka, T. and Tsuzuki, H. (1979). Semi-synthesis of human insulin by trypsin-catalyzed replacement of Ala-B30 by Thr in porcine insulin. *Nature*, **280**, 412–13

61. Wang, S.-S. and Carpenter, F. H. (1969). Kinetics of the tryptic hydrolysis of zinc-free bovine insulin. *J. Biol. Chem.*, **244**, 5537–43

62. Morihara, K, Oka, T. and Tsuzuki, H. (1982/1983). US patent 4,320,196. *Priority*, Apr. 13, 1979. US patent 4,400,465. *Priority*, Apr. 13, 1979

63. Gattner, H.-G., Danho, W. and Naithani, V. K. (1980). Enzyme-catalyzed semisynthesis with insulin derivatives. In Brandenburg, D. and Wollmer, A. (eds.) *Insulin. Chemistry, Structure and Function of Insulin and Related Hormones.* Proceedings of the second International Insulin Symposium. pp. 117–23. (Berlin, New York: Walter de Gruyter)

64. Colletti-Previero, M.-A., Previero, A. and Zuckerkandl, E. (1969). Separation of the proteolytic and esterasic actvities of trypsin by reversible structural modifications. *J. Mol. Biol.*, **39**, 493–501

65. Markussen, J. (1982). US patent 4,343,898. *Priority*, Feb. 11, 1980.

66. Obermeier, R., Ludwig, J. and Seipke, G. (1985). Europäische Patentschrift 0 056 951 B1. *Priority*, Jan. 17, 1981

67. Andresen, F. H. and Balschmidt, P. PCT international publication number WO 82/04069. *Priority*, May 20, 1981

68. Jonczyk, A. and Gattner, H.-G. Deutsches Patentamt Offenlegungsschrift DE 3,129,404 A1. *Priority*, July 25, 1981

69. Markussen, J. and Schaumburg, K. (1983). Reaction mechanism in trypsin catalyzed synthesis of human insulin studied by ^{17}O-NMR spectroscopy. In Blaha, K. and Malon, P. (eds.) *Peptides 1982.* Proceedings of the 17th European Peptide Symposium. pp. 387–94. (Berlin, New York: Walter de Gruyter)

70. Markussen, J. and Vølund, Å. (1983). Kinetics of tryptic transpeptidation of insulins. In Hruby, V. J. ʹand Rich, D. H. (eds.) *Peptides. Structure and Function.* Proceedings of the eighth American Peptide Symposium. pp. 207–10. (Rockford Ill.: Pierce Chemical Company)

71. Markussen, J. and Vølund, Å. (1985). Kinetics of trypsin catalysis in the industrial conversion of porcine insulin to human insulin. In Porter, R. and Clark, S. (eds.) *Enzymes in Organic Synthesis.* Ciba Foundation Symposium 111. pp. 188–203. (London: Pitman)

72. Obermeier, R. and Seipke, G. (1984). Enzyme-catalyzed semisyntheses with porcine insulin. *Process Biochemistry* February, 29–32

73. Jonczyk, A. and Gattner, H.-G. (1981). Eine neue Semisynthese des Humaninsulins. Tryptisch-katalysierte Transpeptidierung von Schweineinsulin mit L-Threonin-tert-butyles-ter. *Hoppe Seyler's Z. Physiol. Chem.,* **362**, 1591–8

74. Offord, R. E. and Rose, K. PCT international publication number WO 83/02772. *Priority,* Feb. 8, 1982

75. Rose, K., De Pury, H. and Offord, R. E. (1983). Rapid preparation of human insulin and insulin analogues in high yields by enzyme-assisted semi-synthesis. *Biochem. J.,* **211**, 671–6

76. Rose, K., Gladstone, J. and Offord, R. E. (1984). A mass-spectrometric investigation of the mechanism of the semisynthetic transformation of pig insulin into an ester of insulin of human sequence. *Biochem. J.,* **220**, 189–96

77. Breddam, K., Widmer, F. and Johansen, J. T. (1981). Carboxypeptidase Y catalyzed C-terminal modification of the B-chain of porcine insulin. *Carlsberg Res. Commun.,* **46**, 361–72

78. Breddam, K., Widmer, F. and Johansen, J. T. Danish patent application 3197 of 1980. *Priority,* Dec. 30, 1980.

79. Breddam, K. and Johansen, J. T. (1984). Semisynthesis of human insulin utilizing chemically modified carboxypeptidase Y. *Carlsberg Res. Commun.,* **49**, 463–72

80. Breddam, K. and Johansen, J. T. Danish patent application 277 of 1982. *Priority,* June 1, 1982

81. Morihara, K., Oka, T., Tsuzuki, H., Tochino, Y. and Kanaya, T. (1980). Achromobacter protease I-catalyzed conversion of porcine insulin into human insulin. *Biochem. Biophys. Res. Commun.,* **92**, 396–402

82. Masaki, T., Nakamura, K., Isono, M. and Soejima, M. (1978). A new proteolytic enzyme from Achromobacter lyticus M497-1. *Agric. Biol. Chem.,* **42**, 1443–5

83. Muneyuki, R., Oka, T. and Morihara, K. (1982). Enzyme immobilization and its application to the process of synthesizing human insulin from porcine insulin. In Shiori, T. (ed.) *Peptide Chemistry 1981.* Proceedings of the Japanese Peptide Symposium. pp. 113–18. (Osaka: Protein Research Foundation)

84. Morihara, K. and Oka, T. (1983). Enzymatic semisynthesis of human insulin by transpeptid-ation method with Achromobacter protease: comparison with the coupling method. In Sakakibara, S. (ed.) *Peptide Chemistry 1982.* Proceedings of the Japanese Peptide Symposium. pp. 231–6. (Osaka: Protein Research Foundation)

85. Soejima, M., Masaki, T., Suzuki, H., Nagaoka, J., Sakata, Y., Shintani, A., Minamii, N., Matsuo, T., Sugiyama, H. and Tokioka, N. Danish patent application 1824 of 1983, *Priority,* Apr. 23, 1982

86. Markussen, J. Jørgensen, K. H., Sørensen, A. R. and Thim, L. (1985). Single chain des-(B30) insulin. Intramolecular crosslinking of insulin by trypsin catalyzed transpeptidation. *Int. J. Pept. Protein Res.,* **26**, 70–7

87. Markussen, J. (1985). Comparative reduction/oxidation studies with single chain des-(B30) insulin and porcine proinsulin. *Int. J. Pept. Protein Res.,* **25**, 431–4

88. Markussen, J., Fiil, N., Thim, L., Norris, K., Voigt, H. O., Ammerer, G. and Hansen, M. T. Danish patent application 2665 of 1984 and 582 of 1985. *Priority,* May 30, 1984

89. Markussen, J. (1984). Semisynthesis of human insulin. In Larner, J. and Pohl, S. (eds.) *Methods in Diabetes Research.* Vol. 1. pp. 403–11. (New York: John Wiley & Sons)

90. Inouye, K., Watanabe, K., Tochino, Y., Kobayashi, M. and Shigeta, Y. (1983). Semisynthesis of human insulin analogues containing a D-amino acid residue in position B24, B25 or B26. In Sakakibara, S. (ed.) *Peptide Chemistry 1982.* Proceedings of the Japanese Peptide Symposium. pp. 277–82. (Osaka: Protein Research Foundation)

91. Gattner, H.-G., Danho, W., Knorr, R., Naithani, V. K. and Zahn, H. (1981). Trypsin catalyzed peptide synthesis: modification of the B-chain C-terminal region of insulin. In Brunfeldt, K. (ed.) *Peptides 1980*. Proceedings of the 16th European Peptide Symposium. pp. 372–7. (Copenhagen: Scriptor)

92. Schlichtkrull, J. (1956). Insulin crystals. I. The minimum mole-fraction of metal in insulin crystals prepared with Zn^{++}, Cd^{++}, Co^{++}, Ni^{++}, Cu^{++}, Mn^{++}, or Fe^{++}. *Acta Chem. Scand.*, **10**, 1455–8

93. Schlichtkrull, J., Brange, J., Christiansen, Aa. H., Hallund, O., Heding, L. G., Jørgensen, K. H., Munkgaard Rasmussen, S., Sørensen, E. and Vølund, Å. (1974). Monocomponent insulin and its clinical implications. *Horm. Metab. Res.*, Suppl Series No. 5, 134–43

94. Bates, R. G. (1954). *Determination of pH. Theory and Practice*. pp. 172–200. (New York, London, Sydney: John Wiley & Sons)

95. Linnet, N. (1970). *pH Measurement in Theory and Practice*. pp. 93–4. (Copenhagen: Radiometer A/S)

96. Gutbezahl, B. and Grunwald, E. (1953). The acidity and basicity scale in the system ethanol-water. The evaluation of degenerate activity coefficients for single ions. *J. Am. Chem. Soc.*, **75**, 565–72

97. Douzou, P. and Balny, C. (1978). Protein fractionation at subzero temperatures. *Adv. Protein Chem.*, **32**, 100–24

98. U.S. Pharmacopoeia USP XX, National Formulary NF XV (1980). pp. 834–5. (Rockville, Maryland: United States Pharmacopoeial Convention Inc.)

99. Walsh, K. A. (1970). In Perlmann, G. E. and Lorand, L. (eds.) *Methods Enzymology*. Vol. XIX, p. 59. (New York: Academic Press)

100. Kostka, V. and Carpenter, F. H. (1964). Inhibition of chymotrypsin activity in crystalline trypsin preparations. *J. Biol. Chem.*, **239**, 1799–1803

101. Robbins, K. C. and Summaria, L. (1970). In Perlmann, G. E. and Lorand, L. (eds.) *Methods Enzymology*. Vol. XIX, pp. 184–6. (New York: Academic Press)

102. Walsh, K. A. and Wilcox, P. E. (1970). In Perlmann, G. E. and Lorand, L. (eds) *Methods Enzymology*. Vol. XIX, pp. 37–8. (New York: Academic Press)

103. Davis, B. J. (1964). Disc electrophoresis II. Method and application to human serum proteins. *Ann. NY Acad. Sci.*, **121**, 404–27

104. Harris, J. I. (1956). Effect of urea on trypsin and alpha-chymotrypsin. *Nature*, **177**, 471–3

105. Erlanger, B. F., Kokowsky, N. and Cohen, W. (1961). The preparation and properties of two new chromogenic substrates of trypsin. *Arch. Biochem. Biophys.*, **95**, 271–8

106. Lazdunski, M. and Delaage, M. (1965). Sur la morphologie des trypsines de porc et de boeuf. Étude des dénaturations reversibles. *Biochem. Biophys. Acta*, **105**, 541–61

107. Wu, H.-L., Kundrot, C. and Bender, M. L. (1982). The denaturation of trypsin. *Biochem. Biophys. Res. Commun.*, **107**, 742–5

108. Inouye, K., Watanabe, K., Tochino, Y., Kobayashi, M. and Shigeta, Y. (1981). Semisynthesis and properties of some insulin analogs. *Biopolymers*, **20**, 1845–58

109. Delaage, M. and Lazdunski, M. (1968). Trypsinogen, trypsin, trypsin-substrate and trypsin-inhibitor complexes in urea solutions. *Eur. J. Biochem.*, **4**, 378–84

110. Baker, E. N., Cutfield, J. F., Cutfield, S. M., Dodson, E. J., Dodson, G. G., Hodgkin, D. C., Hubbard, R. E., Isaacs, N. W., Reynolds, C. D., Sakabe, K., Sakabe, N. and Vijayan, N. M. (1987). The structure of 2Zn pig insulin crystals at 1.5 Å resolution. *Philos. Trans. R. Soc.* (In press)

111. Milthorpe, B. K., Nichol, L. W. and Jeffrey, P. D. (1977). The polymerization pattern of zinc(II)-insulin at pH 7.0. *Biochim. Biophys. Acta*, **495**, 195–202

112. Markussen, J. (1978). Proteolytic degradation of proinsulin and of the intermediate forms: application to synthesis and biosynthesis of insulin. In Baba, S., Kaneko, T. and Yanaihara, N. (eds.) Proceedings of the *Symposium on proinsulin, insulin and C-peptide*. pp. 50–61. (Amsterdam, Oxford, International Congress Series No. 468: Excerpta Medica)

113. Kurjan, J. and Herskowitz, I. (1982). Structure of a yeast pheromone gene (MFα): a putative α-factor precursor contains four tandem copies of mature α-factor. *Cell*, **30**, 933–43

114. Seydoux, F., Yon, J. and Némethy, G. (1969). Hydrophobic interactions of some alcohols with acyl trypsins. *Biochim. Biophys. Acta*, **171**, 145–56

115. Fink, A. L. (1973). The α-chymotrypsin-catalyzed hydrolysis of *N*-acetyl-L-tryptophan *p*-nitrophenyl ester in dimethyl sulfoxide at subzero temperatures. *Biochemistry*, **12**, 1736–42

116. Tanizawa, K. and Bender, M. L. (1974). The application of insolubilized α-chymotrypsin to kinetic studies on the effect of aprotic dipolar organic solvents. *J. Biol. Chem.*, **249**, 2130–4
117. Nilsson, K. and Mosbach, K. (1984). Peptide synthesis in aqueous-organic solvent mixtures with α-chymotrypsin immobilized to tresyl chloride-activated agarose. *Biotechnol. Bioeng.*, **26**, 1146–54
118. Liem, R. K. H. and Scheraga, H. A. (1973). Mechanism of action of thrombin on fibrinogen. III. Partial mapping of the active sites of thrombin and trypsin. *Arch. Biochem. Biophys.*, **158**, 387–95
119. Lobo, A. P., Wos, J. D., Yu, S. M. and Lawson, W. B. (1976). Active site studies of human thrombin and bovine trypsin: peptide substrates. *Arch. Biochem. Biophys.*, **177**, 235–44
120. McRae, B. J., Kurachi, K., Heimark, R. L., Fujikawa, K., Davie, E. W. and Powers, J. C. (1981). Mapping the active sites of bovine thrombin, factor IX_a, factor X_a, factor XI_a, factor XII_a, plasma kallikrein, and trypsin with amino acid and peptide thioesters: development of new sensitive substrates. *Biochemistry*, **20**, 7196–206
121. Barshop, B. A., Wrenn, R. F. and Frieden, C. (1983). Analysis of numerical methods for computer simulation of kinetic processes: development of KINSIM – a flexible, portable system. *Anal. Biochem.*, **130**, 134–45

Tables

Table 1 Physical constants of the L-threonine esters selected for transpeptidation studies

	Melting point (°C)	Optical rotation			pK
		$[\alpha]_D$	c	Solvent	
H-Thr-OMe	64.5–65.5	4.1°	2.5	MeOH	6.8
H-Thr-OBu^t	Oil				
H-Thr-OBu^t, HOAc	55–56	−15.8°	5	H$_2$O	
H-Thr(Bu^t)-OBu^t	Oil				7.2
H-Thr(Bu^t)-OBu^t, HOAc	58–60	−22.2°	5	H$_2$O	
H-Thr-OTmb	94.0–94.5				

Table 2 Comparisons between calculated nominal % water and Karl Fischer (K.F.) analysis. Examples from ref. 65

	Example no.				
	4	6	8	19	*
K.F. analysis (%) (w/v)	42.4	43.9	40.1	20.6	50.7
Nominal % H$_2$O	43.0	43.0	38.4	20.4	50.0
Difference	−0.6	+0.9	+1.7	+0.2	+0.7

*Construed example not reported elsewhere. The solution consisted of: 20 mg insulin, 100 μl 10 M HOAc, 200 μl 2 M Thr-OMe in DMAC, 190 μl H$_2$O and 2 mg trypsin in 25 μl aqueous 0.05 M calcium acetate

Table 3 Comparisons of readings using a glass electrode in non-aqueous solutions, the pH measured after a 100 × dilution in water, and the calculated pH. Based on examples from references 65 and 66 and Table 16

Reference	65				66		Table 16	
Example No.	6	19	29	1	6	9	10	
Organic solvent	HMPA	DMAC	DMAC	DMF	Thr(Buᵗ)-OBuᵗ, HOAc	Thr(Buᵗ)-OBuᵗ, HOAc	Thr(Buᵗ)-OBuᵗ, HOAc	DMAC
H_2O % (w/v), Karl Fischer	45.3	22.0	47.4	39.5	38.0	39.5	53.3	21.7
Glass electrode reading	6.0	6.4	7.7	7.1	5.1	5.7	5.3	7.4
pH after 100 × dilution in water	5.0	4.4	6.9	5.8	4.7	5.0	5.0	5.7
Δ 'pH'	1.0	2.0	0.8	1.3	0.4	0.7	0.3	1.7
Buffer system								
$HOAc/OAc^-$	0.25/1	2.0/1		0.2/1	1/1	0.43/1	0.54/1	0/1
H^+-Thr-OMe/Thr-OMe			0.67/1					1/0
Calculated pH = pK + log B/A	5.3	4.4	7.0	5.4	4.7	5.1	5.0	5.8*

*Calculated using pH = $\frac{1}{2}(pK_1 + pK_2)$

110

Table 4 Corresponding values of specificity q, maximum yield B_{max} and ratio between substrate A and by-product C for concurrent reactions at two sites on substrate A, the product B having a site for the by-product formation

q	B_{max}	A/C (t_{max})
0	0	$(e-1)^{-1}$
0.001	0.0004	0.5819
0.01	0.0037	0.5808
0.1	0.0350	0.5704
1	0.25	0.5
10	0.7153	0.3355
100	0.9454	0.2096
1000	0.9921	0.1441

Table 5 Autolysis of trypsin expressed as the second-order rate constant of autolysis, k_a

Buffer	H_2O (%)	k_a $(h^{-1} mM^{-1})$		
		$12°C$	$25°C$	$38°C$
HOAc/OAc$^-$	20.7	0.055*	1.9	7
1.5/1	25.0	0.055	0.63	9
	30.0	0.013	0.35	15
HOAc/OAc$^-$	20.7	0.25	6	9
0/1	25.0	0.17	0.59	15
	30.0	0.06	0.14	33
H$^+$-Thr-OMe/Thr-OMe	20.7	0.55	5	7
0.5/0.5	25.0	0.31	0.78	14
	30.0	0.15	0.21	32

*Conditions used in the kinetic studies

Conditions
Organic solvent	DMAC
H$_2$O, % nominal	20.7, 25.0, 30.0
Buffer (M/M)	HOAc/OAc$^-$ 1.5/1, 0/1; H$^+$-Thr-OMe/Thr-OMe 0.5/0.5
Threonine ester	1 M Thr-OMe
Temperature (°C)	12, 25, 38
Calcium	3 mM
Substrate	8 mM ~ 5% (w/v) porcine insulin FC
Enzyme	0.2 mM ~ 0.5% (w/v) porcine trypsin TC

Analysis
Sampling (h)	1, 2, 4, 24, 48
Preparation	100-fold dilution in Tris/Ca^{2+} buffer pH 7.8
Method	Photometric using BAPA

Table 6 Yields of HI-OMe (α) and by-products DOI plus DOI-Thr-OMe (β) in coupling reactions. The difference to 100% is DAI plus HI, the latter formed by hydrolysis of HI-OMe

| Ca^{2+} (mM) | t (°C) | Yields (%) | | | |
| | | 24 h | | 96 h | |
		α	β	α	β
2.4	25	74	23	41	58
	37	61	36	55	34
0	25	70	27	40	57
	37	83	4	62	3

Conditions

Organic solvent	BD
H_2O, % nominal	4.8
Buffer (M/M)	HOAc/OAc⁻ 0/1
Threonine ester	1 M Thr-OMe
Temperature (°C)	25, 37
Calcium	0, 2.4 mM
Substrate	8 mM ~ 5% (w/v) DAI
Enzyme	0.2 mM ~ 0.5% (w/v) porcine trypsin TC

Analysis

Sampling (h)	24, 96
Preparation	Acetone precipitation
Method	HPLC, isocratic elution

Table 7 Yields of HI-OMe (α) and by-products DOI plus DOI-Thr-OMe (β) in coupling reactions. The difference to 100% is DAI plus HI

| H_2O (%) | Ca^{2+} (mM) | t (°C) | Yield (%) | | | | | | | |
| | | | 0.5 h | | 1 h | | 2.25 h | | 4 h | |
			α	β	α	β	α	β	α	β
16.6	4	12	84	0	90	1	90	1	91	2
	4	25	92	0	91	1	89	1	89	1
	0	12	55	0	72	1	85	1	89	1
	0	25	39	0	38	0	38	1	38	1
11.8	4	12	81	0	85	1	89	1	89	2
	4	25	85	0	85	1	89	1	74	1
	0	12	48	0	58	1	68	1	67	1
	0	25	31	0	28	0	26	1	23	1

Conditions

Organic solvent	Ethanol
H_2O, % nominal	11.8, 16.6
Buffer (M/M)	HOAc/OAc⁻ 2/1.33
Threonine ester	1.33 M Thr-OMe
Temperature (°C)	12, 25
Calcium	0, 4 mM
Substrate	6.7% (w/v) DAI
Enzyme	0.42% (w/v) porcine trypsin TC

Analysis

Sampling (h)	0.5, 1, 2.25, and 4
Preparation	Acetone precipitation
Method	HPLC, isocratic elution

Table 8 Yields of HI-OMe (α) and DOI plus DOI-Thr-OMe (β) in $2 \times 3 \times 3$ factorial coupling experiment. The difference to 100% is DAI plus HI

Ca^{2+} (mM)	Organic solvent	t (°C)	Yield (%)							
			0.5 h		1 h		2 h		4 h	
			α	β	α	β	α	β	α	β
0	DMAC	12	89	1	92	0	89	1	93	2
		25	95	0	92	0	86	0	85	1
		37	60	1	55	0	45	0	45	1
	EtOH	12	61	1	75	1	79	2	80	2
		25	39	1	37	0	34	0	33	1
		37	3	0	3	0	4	0	5	1
	BD	12	47	1	59	1	72	2	78	4
		25	66	2	73	2	74	4	70	6
		37	28	0	28	0	33	1	30	1
3.8	DMAC	12	92	1	88	1	88	2	89	2
		25	93	2	95	1	90	2	93	3
		37	85	1	90	1	66	1	63	1
	EtOH	12	79	2	83	2	71	3	79	5
		25	83	2	78	2	64	2	69	2
		37	30	1	28	0	21	0	25	0
	BD	12	41	1	47	1	65	2	69	3
		25	73	2	61	2	70	5	73	8
		37	66	2	62	2	63	2	53	2

Conditions
Organic solvent   DMAC, BD, ethanol
H_2O, % nominal   20.9
Buffer (M/M)   HOAc/OAc$^-$ 1.85/1.25
Threonine ester   1.25 M Thr-OMe
Temperature (°C)   12, 25, 37
Calcium   0, 3.8 mM
Substrate   6.15% (w/v) DAI
Enzyme   0.38% (w/v) porcine trypsin TC

Analysis
Sampling (h)   0.5, 1, 2, 4
Preparation   Acetone precipitation
Method   HPLC, isocratic elution

Table 9 Yields of HI-OMe (α), by-products DOI plus DOI-Thr-OMe (β) and specificity (q) in transpeptidation reactions. The difference to 100% is made up of DAI plus HI

H$_2$O (%)	Ca^{2+} (mM)	Trypsin (%)	0.25 h		0.5 h		1 h		2 h		4 h		22 h		q
			α	β	α	β	α	β	α	β	α	β	α	β	
27.1	0	0.1	—	—	6	0	11	0	15	0	11	0	—	—	—
		0.5	28	2	35	3	39	3	42	4	43	3	41	4	27
	2.5	0.1	16	0	20	3	28	2	35	2	42	3	43	4	14
		0.5	41	3	54	5	62	8	74	11	74	12	73	15	26
32.1	0	0.1	9	0	17	1	21	2	25	3	28	6	30	5	20
		0.5	46	6	58	11	67	17	66	26	63	33	—	—	11
	2.5	0.1	14	0	26	2	34	4	51	8	66	11	64	29	14
		0.5	51	8	63	17	66	26	53	44	36	60	—	—	10

Conditions

Organic solvent	DMAC
H$_2$O, % nominal	27.1, 32.1
Buffer (M/M)	H$^+$-Thr-OMe/Thr-OMe 0.5/0.5
Threonine ester	1 M Thr-OMe
Temperature (°C)	37
Calcium	0, 2.5 mM
Substrate	5% (w/v) porcine insulin FC
Enzyme	0.1, 0.5% (w/v) porcine trypsin TC

Analysis

Sampling (h)	0.25, 0.5, 1, 2, 4, 22
Preparation	Acetone precipitation
Method	HPLC, isocratic elution

Table 10 Yields of HI-OMe (α) and by-products DOI plus DOI-Thr-OMe (β) in transpeptidation reactions

		Yield (%)							
		Porcine insulin FC				Porcine insulin MC			
Ca^{2+}	Zn^{2+}	Trypsin TC		TPCK trypsin		Trypsin TC		TPCK trypsin	
(mM)	(mM)	α	β	α	β	α	β	α	β
0	0	48	17	53	35	49	18	49	41
10	0	9	90	9	90	5	94	8	91
0	10	44	12	55	24	43	12	53	28
10	10	15	83	10	89	6	83	13	86

Conditions

Organic solvent	DMAC
H_2O, % nominal	43.3
Buffer (M/M)	HOAc/OAc⁻ 0.67/1
Threonine ester	1 M Thr-OMe
Temperature (°C)	37
Calcium	0, 10 mM
Zinc	0, 10 mM
Substrate	5% (w/v) porcine insulin FC, porcine insulin MC
Enzyme	0.5% (w/v) porcine trypsin TC TPCK treated trypsin

Analysis

Sampling (h)	18
Preparation	Acetone precipitation
Method	HPLC, isocratic elution

Table 11 Yields of HI-OMe in coupling reactions. The difference to 100% is DAI plus HI. By-products DOI and DOI-Thr-OMe are less than 0.7% in all samples. K_e(IM) represents equilibrium constant of the DAI + Thr-OMe $\rightleftharpoons$ HI-OMe + H_2O reaction

Organic solvent	H_2O (%)	Yields (%)								
		4°C			12°C			25°C		
		4 h	24 h	K_e(IM)	4 h	24 h	K_e(IM)	4 h	24 h	K_e(IM)
DMAC	19.8	95	97	340	97	97	340	98	98	540
	13.4	82	93	—	69	83	—	30	31	—
DMF	19.8	97	97	340	97	97	340	97	97	340
	13.4	55	53	—	74	73	—	25	26	—
DMSO	19.8	97	97	340	91	94	—	72	72	—
	13.4	4	4	—	4	4	—	6	5	—
NMP	19.8	96	96	260	92	97	340	86	88	—
	13.4	39	37	—	34	42	—	12	—	—

Conditions
Organic solvent	DMAC, DMF, DMSO, NMP
H_2O, % nominal	13.4, 19.8
Buffer (M/M)	HOAc/OAc⁻ 1.5/1
Threonine ester	1 M Thr-OMe
Temperature (°C)	4, 12, 25
Calcium	2 mM
Substrate	5% (w/v) DAI
Enzyme	0.34% (w/v) porcine trypsin TC

Analysis
Sampling (h)	4, 24
Preparation	Acetone precipitation
Method	HPLC, isocratic elution

Table 12 Yields of HI-OMe (α), DOI plus DOI-Thr-OMe (β) and specificity (q) in transpeptidation reactions

H_2O (%)	HOAc/OAc⁻ (M/M)											
	0.175/0.5			0.25/0.5			0.325/0.5			0.4/0.5		
	α	β	q	α	β	q	α	β	q	α	β	q
46	7	92	1	16	82	1	35	57	2	47	42	7
33	42	4	14	42	4	14	33	2	20	27	3	11
27	7	0	—	7	0	—	9	0	—	7	0	—
21	5	0	—	—	—	—	—	—	—	—	—	—

Conditions

Organic solvent	DMAC
H_2O, % nominal	21, 27, 33, 46
Buffer (M/M)	HOAc/OAc⁻ 0.175/0.5, 0.25/0.5, 0.325/0.5, 0.4/0.5
Threonine ester	0.5 M Thr-OMe
Temperature (°C)	37
Calcium	0 mM
Substrate	2.5% (w/v) porcine insulin FC
Enzyme	0.38% (w/v) porcine trypsin, crystallized once

Analysis

Sampling (h)	18
Preparation	Acetone precipitation
Method	HPLC, isocratic elution

Table 13 Yields of HI-OMe (α), DOI plus DOI-Thr-OMe (β) and specificity (q) in transpeptidation reactions

H_2O (%)	H⁺-Thr-OMe/Thr-OMe (M/M)												HOAc/OAc⁻ (M/M)								
	0/0.5			0.25/0.25			0.4/0.1			0.5/0			0.1/0.5			0.25/0.5			0.5/0.5		
	α	β	q	α	β	q	α	β	q	α	β	q	α	β	q	α	β	q	α	β	q
45																38	52	2	40	13	4
41	13	81	0.7							27	69	2	45	46	3	55	18	6			
37				23	72	1.4	54	37	4	59	16	7	52	9	9						
35	32	55	1.6																		
32.5				62	20	7	38	5	10	27	2	16	22	1	25						
29	23	7	4	23	2	13															
27							11	1	12	8	0	—	8	0	—						

Conditions

Organic solvent	DMAC
H_2O, % nominal	Variable, range 27–45
Buffer (M/M)	HOAc/OAc⁻ 0.1/0.5, 0.25/0.5, 0.5/0.5
	H⁺-Thr-OMe/Thr-OMe 0/0.5, 0.25/0.25, 0.4/0.1, 0.5/0
Threonine ester	0.5 M Thr-OMe
Temperature (°C)	37
Calcium	0 mM
Substrate	2.5% (w/v) porcine insulin FC
Enzyme	0.38% (w/v) porcine trypsin TC

Analysis

Sampling (h)	18
Preparation	Acetone precipitation
Method	HPLC, isocratic elution

Table 14 Yields of HI-OMe (α) and DOI plus DOI-Thr-OMe (β) and specificity (q) in transpeptidation reactions

Time (h)	H_2O (%)	H^+-Thr-OMe/Thr-OMe (M/M)							
		0.75/0.25		1/0					
		27.0		34.3		29.3		25.5	
		α	β	α	β	α	β	α	β
0.5		32	1	49	6	42	2	23	0
2		—	—	70	20	66	7	—	—
4		32	1	63	33	71	9	23	0
q		37		12		31		—	

Time (h)	H_2O (%)	HOAc/OAc$^-$ (M/M)												
		0.25/1								0.5/1					
		42.8		37.9		32.8		27.9		41.4		36.4		31.4	
		α	β	α	β	α	β	α	β	α	β	α	β	α	β
0.5		—	—	—	—	48	4	39	1	—	—	44	5	41	2
2		51	41	64	26	72	14	52	3	58	33	68	16	64	7
4		32	65	53	43	71	22	56	4	49	44	67	25	73	10
q		4		7		18		66		5		14		30	

Conditions

Organic solvent	DMAC
H_2O, % nominal	Variable, range 25.5–42.8
Buffer (M/M)	HOAc/OAc$^-$ 0.25/1, 0.5/1
	H^+-Thr-OMe/Thr-OMe 0.75/0.25, 1/0
Threonine ester	1 M Thr-OMe
Temperature (°C)	37
Calcium	3 mM
Substrate	5% (w/v) porcine insulin FC
Enzyme	0.5% (w/v) porcine trypsin TC

Analysis

Sampling (h)	0.5, 2, 4
Preparation	Acetone precipitation
Method	HPLC, isocratic elution

Table 15 Yields of HO-OMe (α) and DOI plus DOI-Thr-OMe (β) in transpeptidation reactions. The difference to 100% is DAI ($+$ HI $+$ PI).

HOAc/OAc⁻ (M/M)	H₂O (%)	12°C								18°C							
		4 h		27 h		48 h		q	$K_e(IM)$	4 h		27 h		48 h		q	$K_e(IM)$
		α	β	α	β	α	β			α	β	α	β	α	β		
1/1	23.6	47	0	90	2	93	3	250	300	59	1	92	4	90	7	150	300
	21.1	36	0	87	1	91	1	300	*	57	0	91	2	88	2	300	*
	19.8	34	0	83	1	89	1	300	*	45	0	79	1	83	1	400	*
1.25/1	22.1	41	0	90	2	94	3	200	400	59	1	93	3	89	5	200	300
	19.6	33	0	83	0	87	1	500	*	47	0	84	1	81	1	400	*
	18.4	32	0	72	0	82	0	†	*	41	0	62	0	62	0	†	*
1.5/1	20.7	37	0	88	1	93	2	300	200	58	0	91	2	88	3	300	*
	18.2	32	0	76	0	82	0	†	*	42	0	67	0	64	0	†	*
	17.0	27	0	61	0	66	0	†	*	32	0	46	0	40	0	†	*

* Equilibrium not established; trypsin inactivation and/or slow reactions
† Specificity q is high, but inaccessible to quantitation

Conditions

Organic solvent	DMAC
H₂O, % nominal	Variable, range 17.0–23.6
Buffer (M/M)	HOAc/OAc⁻ 1/1, 1.25/1, 1.5/1
Threonine ester	1 M Thr-OMe
Temperature (°C)	12, 18
Calcium	3 mM
Substrate	5% (w/v) porcine insulin FC
Enzyme	0.5% (w/v) porcine trypsin TC

Analysis

Sampling (h)	4, 27, 48
Preparation	Isopropyl alcohol precipitation
Method	HPLC, isocratic elution

Table 16 Yields of HI-OMe (α) and DOI plus DOI-Thr-OMe (β) in transpeptidation reactions. The difference to 100% is made up of DAI (+ PI + HI). The large variations in K_e(IM) estimates are possibly due to HI formation

Buffer (M/M)	H_2O (%)	Yields (%) 65 h α	65 h β	89 h α	89 h β	113 h α	113 h β	q	$K_e(IM)$	
H$^+$-Thr-OMe/	28.4	50	49	37	60	—	—	> 6	200–800	*
Thr-OMe	26.7	72	24	—	—	—	—	>̇10	300	*
0.5/0.5	25.2	66	30	—	—	—	—	> 8	200	*
	23.9	84	15	80	17	—	—	>̇30	300–1100	*
	22.7	81	16	80	20	77	19	>̇20	300	*
H$^+$-Thr-OMe	25.5	86	13	82	14	—	—	>̇30	300–1200	*
Thr-OMe	24.0	86	11	87	9	—	—	>̇30	300–400	*
1/0	22.7	88	9	—	—	—	—	>̇40	400	*
	21.5	81	2	83	1	83	2	>̇90		†
	20.4	92	2	—	—	93	3	>150		†
HOAc/OAc$^-$	22.6	92	5	92	2	88	8	>̇70	400	*
0.5/1	21.3	97	2	93	3	93	4	>225	300–1200	*
	20.2	63	0	63	0	63	0	‡		†
	19.1	20	0	25	0	24	0	‡		†
	18.1	16	0	17	0	13	0	‡		†
HOAc/OAc$^-$	19.8	96	2	—	—	95	0	>200	500	
1/1	18.7	90	1	91	0.5	91	1	>250		†
	17.6	81	0	81	0	83	0	‡		†
	16.7	22	0	27	0	27	0	‡		†
	15.9	31	0	30	0	30	0	‡		†
HOAc/OAc$^-$	17.0	84	0	87	0	87	0	‡		†
1.5/1	16.0	71	0	71	0	70	0	‡		†
	15.1	42	0	41	0	42	0	‡		†
	14.3	16	0	29	0	22	0	‡		†
	13.6	17	0	20	0	15	0	‡		†

* Precipitation during reactions
† Equilibrium not established, trypsin inactivation and/or slow reactions
‡ Specificity q is high, but inaccessible to quantitation

Conditions
Organic solvent   DMAC
H$_2$O, % nominal   Variable, range 13.6–28.4
Buffer (M/M)   HOAc/OAc$^-$ 1.5/1, 1/1, 0.5/1
                H$^+$-Thr-OMe/Thr-OMe 1/0, 0.5/0.5
Threonine ester   1 M Thr-OMe
Temperature (°C)   12
Calcium   3 mM
Substrate   5% (w/v) porcine insulin FC
Enzyme   0.5% (w/v) porcine trypsin TC

Analysis
Sampling (h)   65, 89, 113
Preparation   Acetone precipitation
Method   HPLC, isocratic elution

Table 17 Yields of HI-OMe (α) and DOI plus DOI-Thr-OMe (β) and specificity (q) in transpeptidation reactions

	23°C								31°C							
HOAc/OAc⁻ (M/M)	0.7/1				1/1				0.7/1				1/1			
Time — H$_2$O (%)	27.8		25.3		26.1		23.6		27.8		25.3		26.1		23.6	
h	α	β	α	β	α	β	α	β	α	β	α	β	α	β	α	β
4	76	4	76	3	76	3	75	2	83	8	77	4	79	4	61	2
24	73	21	81	11	82	13	87	8	80	16	84	5	84	4	66	2
48	62	35	78	18	74	22	86	10	79	16	84	5	83	6	65	2
q	40		79		65		104		28		40		42		48	

	37°C							
HOAc/OAc⁻ (M/M)	0.7/1				1/1			
Time — H$_2$O, %	27.8		25.3		26.1		23.6	
h	α	β	α	β	α	β	α	β
4	56	3	35	1	36	1	19	0
24	56	2	37	1	35	1	20	0
q	28		43		44		—	

Conditions

Organic solvent	DMAC
H$_2$O, % nominal	23.6, 26.1, 25.3, 27.8
Buffer (M/M)	HOAc/OAc⁻ 0.7, 1/1
Threonine ester	1 M Thr-OMe
Temperature (°C)	23 (ambient), 31, 37
Calcium	3 mM
Substrate	5% (w/v) porcine insulin FC
Enzyme	0.5% (w/v) porcine trypsin TC

Analysis

Sampling (h)	4, 24, 48
Preparation	Isopropyl alcohol precipitation
Method	HPLC, isocratic elution

Table 18 Yields of HI-OMe (α), by-products DOI plus DOI-Thr-OMe (β), specificity q and equilibrium constant K_e(IM) at varying concentrations of water and Thr-OMe, assuming equilibrium has been established after transpeptidation

	7°C					12°C				
H_2O (%)	29.4	23.8	20.0	17.2	13.5	29.4	23.8	20.0	17.2	13.5
Thr-OMe (M)	1.5	1.6	1.67	1.71	1.78	1.5	1.6	1.67	1.71	1.78
Enzyme (%)	0.5	0.4	0.33	0.29	0.22	0.5	0.4	0.33	0.29	0.22
Yields										
3.5 h α	65	58	41	30	10	77	78	51	25	9
β	8	4	1	0	0	12	5	2	0	0
24 h α	79	88	91	62	11	79	84	93	57	9
β	12	6	4	0	0	13	12	6	0	0
q	14	22	90	†	†	16	33	80	†	†
K_e(IM)	95	120	120	*	*	110	170	600	*	*

* Equilibrium not established
† Specificity q is high, but inaccessible to quantitation

Conditions
Organic solvent	DMAC
H_2O, % nominal	29.4, 23.8, 20.0, 17.2, 13.5
Buffer, ratio	H^+-Thr-OMe/Thr-OMe 0/1
Threonine ester	1.5, 1.6, 1.67, 1.71, 1.78 M Thr-OMe
Temperature (°C)	7, 12
Calcium	3 mM
Substrate	5% (w/v) porcine insulin FC
Enzyme	Variable, range 0.22–0.5% (w/v) porcine trypsin TC

Analysis
Sampling (h)	3.5, 24
Preparation	Acetone precipitation
Method	HPLC, isocratic elution

Table 19 Yields of HI-OMe (α) and DOI plus DOI-Thr-OMe (β), specificity (q), and equilibrium constant K_e(IM) in transpeptidation reactions

Time (h)	Temperature					
	$-18°C$		$50°C$		$60°C$	
	α	β	α	β	α	β
4	20	0	24	4	10	1
24	67	1	28	4	*	
120	89	2	*		*	
q	330		7		11	
K_e(IM)	150		†		†	

* Precipitations in test tubes
† Enzyme destroyed before establishment of equilibrium

Conditions
Organic solvent   DMAC
H_2O, % nominal   35
Buffer (M/M) H^+-Thr-OMe/Thr-OMe 0.62/0.62
Threonine ester   1.24 M Thr-OMe
Temperature (°C) -18, 50, 60
Calcium   3 mM
Substrate   6.2% (w/v) porcine insulin FC
Enzyme   0.62% (w/v) porcine trypsin TC

Analysis
Sampling (h)   4, 24, 120
Preparation   Acetone precipitation
Method   HPLC, isocratic elution

Table 20 Yields of HI-OMe (α) and DOI + DOI-Thr-OMe (β) and specificity (q) in transpeptidation reactions

H_2O (%)	Temperature					
	$-10°C$		$6°C$		$30°C$	
	α	β	α	β	α	β
54.9	*		—	—	—	—
44.8	64	1	41	54	6	94
q	103		3		~ 0	
17.4	35	0	64	0	12	0
9.4	0	0	0	0	0	0

* Solidified at $-10°C$

Conditions
Organic solvent   DMAC
H_2O, % nominal   9.4, 17.4, 44.8, 54.9
Buffer (M/M) $HOAc/OAc^-$ 1/1
Threonine ester   1 M Thr-OMe
Temperature (°C) -10, 6, 30
Calcium   3 mM
Substrate   5% (w/v) porcine insulin FC
Enzyme   0.5% (w/v) porcine trypsin TC

Analysis
Sampling (h)   72
Preparation   Acetone precipitation
Method   HPLC, isocratic elution

123

Table 21 Yields of HI-OR (α) and DOI plus DOI-Thr-OR (β) in transpeptidation reactions. Specificity q is calculated from best rate estimates, and K_e from 120h data

Thr-OR	Thr-OEt				Thr-OMse				Thr(Bu^t)-OBu^t			
Thr-OR (M)	1.0	1.11	1.22	1.33	0.25	0.28	0.31	0.33	0.5	0.55	0.61	0.67
HOAc/OAc$^-$ (M/M)	1.5/1	1.67/1.11	1.83/1.22	2/1.33	0.5/0.25	0.56/0.28	0.62/0.31	0.66/0.33	1/0.5	1.11/0.55	1.22/0.61	1.34/0.67
H$_2$O (%)	16.0	17.6	19.1	20.9	25.4	28.0	30.4	33.2	21.3	23.6	25.6	27.9
Yields												
3.5h α	4	15	18	55	28	52	32	43	29	41	58	58
β	0	0	0	2	0	0	0	2	0	0	0	0
24h α	28	64	65	83	87	84	73	69	92	90	82	81
β	0	0	1	11	4	6	11	20	4	5	12	12
120h α	49	92	87	73	73	71	50	49	84	81	58	58
β	0	4	9	23	19	21	41	46	12	15	38	37
q	∞	150	70	50	50	100	25	20	90	110	50	50
K_e	*	200	200	150	500	500	300	500	500	500	300	250

* Equilibrium not established

Conditions

Organic solvent	DMAC
H$_2$O, % nominal	variable, 16.0–27.9
Buffer, ratio	HOAc/OAc$^-$, 1.5/1, 2/1
Threonine ester	1–1.33 M Thr-OEt; 0.25–0.33 M Thr-OMse; 0.5–0.67 M Thr(Bu^t)-OBu^t
Temperature (°C)	12
Calcium	3 mM
Substrate	5% (w/v) porcine insulin FC
Enzyme	0.5% (w/v) porcine trypsin TC

Analysis

Sampling (h)	3.5, 24, 120
Preparation	Acetone precipitation
Method	HPLC, gradient elution

124

Table 22 Yields of HI-OMe (α) and DOI plus DOI-Thr-OMe (β) and specificity (q) in transpeptidation reactions. K_e(IM) values are minimum values due to hydrolysis of HI-OMe to HI which is accounted for as DAI

Zn^{2+} (mM)	Time (h)	$\dfrac{H^+\text{-}Thr\text{-}OMe}{Thr\text{-}OMe}$ (M/M)	24.1 1.25/0 α	24.1 1.25/0 β	25.9 0.93/0.31 α	25.9 0.93/0.31 β	27.7 0.62/0.62 α	27.7 0.62/0.62 β	29.4 0.31/0.93 α	29.4 0.31/0.93 β	30.5 0.125/1.125 α	30.5 0.125/1.125 β
0	0.25		19	1	27	4	31	4	34	7	38	12
	0.5		37	3	46	5	—	—	—	—	—	—
	1		54	4	58	10	61	16	57	29	48	40
	2		68	9	70	19	—	—	—	—	30	64
	4		74	14	64	30	50	46	28	70	13	84
	24		71	19	56	43	—	—	—	—	—	—
		q	21		13		9		6		4	
		K_e(IM)	>80		>640		>150		>180		>70	
6	0.25		28	1	28	2	33	4	41	9	40	14
	0.5		41	3	44	5	—	—	—	—	—	—
	1		55	6	59	9	59	17	56	32	47	42
	2		69	9	69	18	—	—	—	—	—	—
	4		74	14	66	28	49	46	24	73	14	83
	24		73	18	53	39	—	—	—	—	—	—
		q	22		13		9		6		4	
		K_e(IM)	>90		>190		>120		>100		>63	

Conditions

Organic solvent	DMAC
H_2O, % nominal	24.1, 25.9, 27.7, 29.4, 30.5
Buffer (M/M)	H^+-Thr-OMe/Thr-OMe 1.25/0, 0.93/0.31, 0.62/0.62, 0.31/0.93, 0.125/1.125
Threonine ester	1.25 M Thr-OMe
Temperature (°C)	37
Calcium	3 mM
Zinc	0, 6 mM
Substrate	6.25% (w/v) porcine insulin FC
Enzyme	0.63% (w/v) porcine trypsin TC

Analysis

Sampling (h)	0.25, 0.5, 1, 2, 4, 24
Preparation	Acetone precipitation
Method	HPLC, isocratic elution

125

Table 23 Yields of HI-OMe (α) and DOI-Thr-OMe (β) and specificity (q) in transpeptidation reactions in acetic acid and propionic acid buffers

Time (h)	H₂O (%)	HOAc/OAc⁻ (M/M)											
		0.5/1						0.73/1					
		31.4		28.9		26.4		30.1		27.6		25.1	
		α	β	α	β	α	β	α	β	α	β	α	β
4		73	10	65	5	37	2	62	4	54	0	29	1
24		75	11	65	5	39	2	62	5	53	2	29	1
q		16		22		23		25		38		34	

Time (h)	H₂O (%)	HOPr/OPr⁻ (M/M)											
		0.5/1						0.73/1					
		28.8		26.3		23.8		27.1		24.6		22.1	
		α	β	α	β	α	β	α	β	α	β	α	β
4		61	8	60	4	36	1	69	5	42	1	27	1
24		76	12	66	5	39	1	70	6	46	2	27	1
q		13		20		45		25		31		32	

Conditions

Organic solvent	DMAC
H₂O, % nominal	Variable, range 22.1–31.4
Buffer (M/M)	HOAc/OAc⁻ 0.5/1, 0.73/1
	HOPr/OPr⁻ 0.5/1, 0.73/1
Threonine ester	1 M Thr-OMe
Temperature (°C)	37
Calcium	3 mM
Substrate	5% (w/v) porcine insulin FC
Enzyme	0.5% (w/v) porcine trypsin TC

Analysis

Sampling (h)	4, 24
Preparation	Isopropyl alcohol precipitation
Method	HPLC, isocratic elution

Table 24 Yields of HI-OMe (α), DOI (β_1), DOI-Thr-OMe (β_2), and the sum of DOI and DOI-Thr-OMe (β) in coupling reactions. K_e(IM), K_e(DM), and q have been estimated where data permitted calculation

	DMAC, 1 M Thr-OMe, HOAc/OAc⁻ 0/1						DMF, 1 M Thr-OMe, HOAc/OAc⁻ 0/1					
H_2O (%)	27.1		20.7		18.7		27.1		20.7		18.7	
Temp. (°C)	12	22	12	−22	12	−22	12	−22	12	−22	12	−22
	α β	α β	α β	α β	α β	α β	α β	α β	α β	α β	α β	α β
	92 5	86 0	98 0	55 0	99 0	— —	56 41 (β₁ 3, β₂ 38)	98 1	98 0	93 0	98 1	83 0
q	>70	—	—	—	—	—	>6	—	—	—	—	—
K_e(IM)	450	100†	600	15*	1000	—	300	1500	600	150*	1000	—
K_e(DM)	—	—	—	—	—	—	200	—	—	—	—	—

	THF, 0.75 M Thr-OMe, HOAc/OAc⁻ 0.25/0.75						Acetone, 1 M Thr-OMe, HOAc/OAc⁻ 0/1					
H_2O (%)	27.1		20.7		18.7		27.1		20.7		18.7	
Temp. (°C)	12	−22	12	−22	12	−22	12	−22	12	−22	12	−22
	α β	α β	α β	α β	α β	α β	α β	α β	α β	α β	α β	α β
	56 36 (β₁ 9, β₂ 27)	91 1	52 43 (β₁ 12, β₂ 31)	88 2	61 35 (β₁ 7, β₂ 28)	91 1	68 26 (β₁ 4, β₂ 22)	92 1	55 42 (β₁ 6, β₂ 36)	89 0	31 64 (β₁ 8, β₂ 56)	91 2
q	>5	250	>4	100	>6	250	>8	250	>5	—	>2	130
K_e(IM)	140	230	160	130	210‡	160‡	170	200	210†	90†	65†	130†
K_e(DM)	60	—	40	—	55	—	80	—	70	—	70	—

* Equilibrium may not have been established
† Precipitation in test tubes during reaction
‡ Solutions turbid from start of reaction

Conditions
Organic solvent	DMAC, DMF, THF, acetone
H_2O, % nominal	18.7, 20.7, 27.1
Buffer (M/M)	HOAc/OAc⁻ 0/1, 0.25/0.75
Threonine ester	1 M and 0.75 M Thr-OMe
Temperature (°C)	−22, 12
Calcium	2 mM
Substrate	5% (w/v) DAI
Enzyme	0.34% (w/v) porcine trypsin TC

Analysis
Sampling (h)	24
Preparation	Acetone precipitation
Method	HPLC isocratic elution

Table 25 Yields of HI-OMe (α) and DOI plus DOI-Thr-OMe (β) and specificity (q) in transpeptidation reactions

	Methanol				Ethanol				Ethylene glycol									
H⁺-Thr-OMe/Thr-OMe (M/M)	1.23/0		0.94/0.47		1.23/0		0.94/0.47		1.23/0		0.94/0.47		0.76/0.76		0.55/1.11		0.43/1.30	
H₂O (%)	31.4		24.0		33.9		25.9		31.4		24.0		19.5		14.1		11.0	
Time (h)	α	β	α	β	α	β	α	β	α	β	α	β	α	β	α	β	α	β
4	4	96	8	92	47	45	39	58	31	10	29	13	37	7	46	3	50	1
69	3	97	2	98	0	100	0	100	3	95	0	100	1	99	7	67	11	48
q	—		—		>3		>3		4		3		7		10		19	
Comments	*		*		†		†		‡				†		†		†	

	Glycerol										Acetone		THF	
H⁺-Thr-OMe/Thr-OMe (M/M)	1.23/0		0.94/0.47		0.76/0.76		0.55/1.11		0.43/1.30		1.23/0		0.31/0.93	
HOAC/OAc⁻ (M/M)														
H₂O (%)	31.4		24.0		19.5		14.1		11.0		31.4		31.4	
	α	β	α	β	α	β	α	β	α	β	α	β	α	β
4	18	2	17	0	11	0	3	0	7	1	50	45	77	8
69	31	23	23	23	10	21	16	15	7	18	8	86	24	61
q	13		12		—		**		**		>4		22	
Comments							**		**		**			

* Reaction rate too high to estimate q
† Unknown peak eluting after DOI-Thr-OMe is possibly DOI-OEt. Unknown peak included in β
‡ Shoulder on porcine insulin peak is possibly DAI-O-CH₂-CH₂-OH, accounted for as unconverted PI (100 − α − β)
** Shoulder on porcine insulin peak is possibly DAI-OCH₂-CHOH-CH₂OH, accounted for as unconverted PI (100 − α − β)

Conditions

Organic solvent	MeOH, EtOH, ethylene glycol, acetone, glycerol, THF
H₂O, % nominal	Variable, range 11.0–31.4
Buffer, ratio	Ht-Thr-OMe/Thr-OMe 1/0, 2/1, 1/1, 1/2, 1/3; HOAc/OAc⁻ 1/3
Threonine ester	Variable, range 0.92–1.73 M Thr-OMe
Temperature (°C)	12
Calcium	3 mM
Substrate	5% (w/v) porcine insulin FC
Enzyme	0.5% (w/v) porcine trypsin TC

Analysis

Sampling (h)	4, 69
Preparation	Acetone precipitation

Table 26 Yields of HI(Bu^t)-OBu^t (α), DOI plus DOI-Thr(Bu^t)-OBu^t (β) and unknown, possibly DAI-O-(CH$_2$)$_4$-OH (γ) in transpeptidation reactions

	NaCl precipitation						Acetone precipitation								
Temp. (°C)	37*			12†			37*			28.5‡			20		
Time (h)	α	β	γ	α	β	γ	α	β	γ	α	β	γ	α	β	γ
0.5	55	3	3	3	0	0	57	4	3	31	1	1	14	0	0
1	76	8	3	8	0	1	78	11	1	45	2	1	23	1	0
2	—	—	—	—	—	—	69	28	0	65	9	0	—	—	—
18	39	51	1	32	3	2	55	42	0	78	16	0	52	6	0
24	42	57	1	56	9	2	24	74	1	55	43	0	70	27	0
Specificity q	21			13			23			16			14		
K_e(IB)	—			**			70			80			65		

* Clear solution after 1.5 h reaction time at 37°C
† Reaction in suspension for 24 h
‡ Clear solution after 5 h reaction time at 28.5°C
** Equilibrium not established in suspension

Conditions

Organic solvent	BD
H$_2$O, % nominal	4.8
Buffer (M/M)	H$^+$-Thr(Bu^t)-OBu^t/Thr(Bu^t)-OBu^t 0.95/0
Threonine ester	0.95 M Thr(Bu^t)-OBu^t
Temperature (°C)	12, 20, 28.5, 37
Calcium	2.4 mM
Substrate	4.8% (w/v) porcine insulin MC
Enzyme	0.48% (w/v) porcine trypsin TC

Analysis

Sampling (h)	0.5, 1, 2, 18, 24
Preparation	Acetone precipitation, NaCl precipitation
Method	HPLC, gradient elution

Table 27 Yields of HI(Buᵗ)-OBuᵗ (α), DOI (β_1), and DOI-Thr(Buᵗ)-OBuᵗ (β_2) in transpeptidation reactions

Temperature (°C)	*12*						*26*								
H_2O (%)	*23.8*						*20.9*			*23.8*					
HOAc/OAc⁻ (M/M)				*4/2*			*0.77/2.31*						*4/2*		
H⁺-Thr(Buᵗ)-OBuᵗ/ Thr(Buᵗ)-OBᵗ (M/M)	*0.83/1.67*									*0.83/1.67*					
	α	β_1	β_2	α	β_1	β_2	α	β_1	β_2	α	β_1	β_2	α	β_1	β_2
2	90	1	2	65	0	1	78	11	6	74	14	8	79	7	1
4	89	5	2	75	5	0	65	17	13	55	22	20	79	13	2
24	63	12	22	69	20	6	27	14	58	30	18	50	67	21	7
48	50	19	29	20*	10	70	22	7	68	19*	11	70	68	20	8
Specificity q	70			80			15			12			23		

* Peak of DAI (+ PI) not integrated

Conditions

Organic solvent	Thr(Buᵗ)-OBuᵗ
H_2O, % nominal	20.9, 23.8
Buffer (M/M)	HOAc/OAc⁻ 0.77/2.31, 4/2
	H⁺-Thr(Buᵗ)-OBuᵗ/Thr(Buᵗ)-OBuᵗ 0.83/1.67
Threonine ester	2 M, 2.31 M, 2.5 M Thr(OBuᵗ)-OBuᵗ
Temperature (°C)	12, 26
Calcium	3 mM
Substrate	6% (w/v) porcine insulin FC
Enzyme	0.4% (w/v) porcine trypsin TC

Analysis

Sampling (h)	2, 4, 24, 48
Preparation	Acetone precipitation
Method	HPLC, gradient elution

Table 28 Yields of HI-OMe (α) and DOI plus DOI-Thr-OMe (β) in transpeptidation reactions in urea solutions

Temp. (°C)	HOAc/OAc⁻ (M/M)	H₂O (%)	Yields (%)			
			4 h		24 h	
			α	β	α	β
4	1/1	60	3	1	5	2
		51	4	0	6	2
	1.25/1	58	3	1	4	2
		50	4	0	6	0
	1.5/1	57	3	1	5	3
		49	4	0	6	0
12	1/1	60	3	1	5	6
		51	4	0	6	7
	1.25/1	58	4	1	5	6
		50	5	1	6	3
	1.5/1	57	3	1	5	5
		49	5	0	4	1

Conditions

Organic solvent	Urea
H₂O, % nominal	Variable, range 49–60
Buffer (M/M)	HOAc/OAc⁻ 1/1, 1.25/1, 1.5/1
Threonine ester	1 M Thr-OMe
Temperature (°C)	4, 12
Calcium	4 mM
Substrate	6% (w/v) porcine insulin FC
Enzyme	0.6% (w/v) porcine trypsin TC

Analysis

Sampling (h)	4, 24
Preparation	NaCl/HCl precipitation
Method	HPLC, isocratic elution

Table 29 Yields of HI-OMe (α), DOI (β_1) and DOI-Thr-OMe (β_2) in transpeptidation reactions in acetamide. Specificity q, equilibrium constants K_e(IM) and K_e(DM) have been estimated from data

Temp. (°C)	HOAc/OAc⁻ (M/M)	H₂O (%)	Yields (%)									q	K_e(IM)†	K_e(DM)
			4 h		24 h			48 h					
			α	β*	α	β_1	β_2	α	β_1	β_2			
12	1/1	42	19	—	45	*	18	37	11	34	4	60	70
		40	27	—	51	1	23	43	4	42	7	90	250
		35	24	—	58	*	7	59	4	16	15	50	80
	1.25/1	41	16	—	45	*	14	41	9	28	7	40	70
		39	24	—	54	*	16	46	7	30	9	60	90
		35	29	—	62	*	9	59	4	21	14	70	100
	1.5/1	40	11	—	38	*	4	44	6	14	6	30	50
		38	17	—	49	*	7	51	5	18	9	40	80
		34	22	—	58	*	6	60	3	14	16	50	90
21	1/1	42	36	—	33	8	46	14	17	63	3	50	90
		40	42	—	42	3	40	27	6	61	6	100	250
		35	57	—	48	*	44	25	9	60	9	80	130
	1.25/1	41	31	—	47	*	32	26	14	49	6	50	80
		39	35	—	57	*	21	47	7	32	11	70	100
		35	41	—	62	1	15	58	4	21	18	70	100
	1.5/1	40	22	—	49	*	14	44	8	25	10	40	70
		38	17	—	34	2	4	35	3	8	18	14	60
		34	27	—	43	*	2	47	*	3	90	16	—

* Peaks not integrated

† K_e(IM) calculated assuming equilibrium has been established. Unconverted porcine insulin may be present and accounted for as DAI

Conditions

Organic solvent	Acetamide
H₂O, % nominal	Variable, range 34–42
Buffer	HOAc/OAc⁻ 1/1, 1.25/1, 1.5/1
Threonine ester	1 M Thr-OMe
Temperature (°C)	12, 21
Calcium	4 mM
Substrate	6% (w/v) porcine insulin FC
Enzyme	0.6% (w/v) porcine trypsin TC

Analysis

Sampling (h)	4, 24, 48
Preparation	NaCl/HCl precipitation
Method	HPLC, isocratic elution

Table 30 Yields of HI-OMe (α), DOI (β_1), and DOI-Thr-OMe (β_2) in transpeptidation reactions in polyethylene glycol. Specificity q and equilibrium constants $K_e(IM)$ and $K_e(DM)$ have been estimated from data

Temp. (°C)	HOAc/OAc⁻ (M/M)	H₂O (%)	Yields (%)									q	$K_e(IM)$†	$K_e(DM)$
			4 h			24 h			48 h					
			α	β_1	β_2	α	β_1	β_2	α	β_1	β_2			
12	0.6/1	34.0	21	1	2	38	8	33	25	11	44	3	25	80
	0.8/1	33.5	14	1	2	26	2	23	21	9	44	3	15	90
	1/1	32.9	14	1	2	25	3	27	15	7	32	3	6	80
	1.25/1	32.1	12	1	1	35	0	4	31	8	24	4	15	50
	1.5/1	31.4	9	0	0	—	*	—	31	4	11	7	10	50
	1.4/1	31.8	16	1	2	—	*	—	29	12	33	3	20	50
	1.7/1	31.0	17	2	2	—	*	—	27	8	32	4	14	70
	2/1	30.2	6	1	0	5	0	1	30	4	8	6	9	30
21	0.6/1	34.0	15	1	3	13	5	29	10	10	43	2	5	80
	0.8/1	33.5	24	2	7	5	9	69	5	13	67	4	6	100
	1/1	32.9	17	1	3	11	4	31	10	12	42	3	5	60
	1/1	32.9	23	1	5	—	*	—	16	7	58	2	15	150
	1.25/1	32.1	30	2	8	—	*	—	12	13	56	5	11	80
	1.5/1	32.4	22	2	4	39	3	41	26	11	42	3	20	70
	1.4/1	31.8	9	1	1	—	*	—	12	13	44	1	7	60
	1.7/1	31.0	37	3	9	—	*	—	20	11	44	4	25	70
	2/1	30.2	25	1	4	—	*	—	41	5	14	9	17	50

* Analyses lost

† $K_e(IM)$ calculated assuming equilibrium has been established. Unconverted porcine insulin may be present and accounted for as DAI

Conditions

Organic solvent	Polyethylene glycol (Macrogol 4000)
H₂O, % nominal	Variable, range 30.2–34.0
Buffer (M/M)	HOAc/OAc⁻ variable, range 0.6/1–2/1
Threonine ester	1 M Thr-OMe
Temperature (°C)	12, 21
Calcium	4 mM
Substrate	6% (w/v) porcine insulin FC
Enzyme	0.6% (w/v) porcine trypsin TC

Analysis

Sampling (h)	4, 24, 48
Preparation	NaCl/HCl precipitation
Method	HPLC, isocratic elution

Table 31   Yield of HI-OMe (α), DOI (β_1) and DOI-Thr-OMe (β_2) in transpeptidation reactions in acetamide plus additions of other organic compounds

Temp. (°C)	Added organic compound	% (w/v)	H_2O (%)	24 h α	24 h β_1	24 h β_2	48 h α	48 h β_1	48 h β_2	168 h α	168 h β_1	168 h β_2	q	$K_e(IM)$‡	$K_e(DM)$
4	None		31.4							65	2	7	14	40	60
	Phenol	20	25.1							18	0	0			
	Phenol	30	22.0							5	0	0			
	GuCl*	10	28.3							6	0	0			
	Ethanol	10	28.3							59	1	6	14	25	90
	DMAC	10	28.3							62	1	5	17	30	80
	PEG†	10	28.3							74	2	11	14	90	86
	PEG	20	25.1							70	1	7	17	44	100
	PEG	30	22.0							73	1	8	17	50	100
12	None		31.4	44	1	3	48	1	5				15	18	90
	Phenol	10	28.3	21	0	1	23	0	1						
	Phenol	20	25.1	4	0	0	5	0	0						
	Phenol	30	22.0	2	0	0	3	0	0						
	GuCl*	10	28.3	0	0	0	0	0	0						
	Ethanol	10	28.3	23	0	1	29	1	2						
	DMAC	10	28.3	39	1	3	41	1	3				13	12	50
	PEG†	10	28.3	42	1	4	49	1	7				11	17	110
	PEG	20	25.1	52	1	5	58	2	8				13	25	60
	PEG	30	22.0	61	1	7	64	2	12				8	35	70

* Guanidinium hydrochloride
† Polyethylene glycol 4000
‡ Assuming equilibrium has been established

Conditions

Organic solvent	Acetamide + addition of other organic compounds
H_2O, % nominal	Variable, range 22–31.4
Buffer (M/M)	HOAc/OAc$^-$ 1.63/1
Threonine ester	1 M Thr-OMe
Temperature (°C)	4, 12
Calcium	3 mM
Substrate	5% (w/v) porcine insulin FC
Enzyme	0.5% (w/v) porcine trypsin TC

Analysis

Sampling (h)	24, 48, 168
Preparation	NaCl/HCl precipitation
Method	HPLC, isocratic elution

134

Table 32 Residual DAI $(100 - \alpha)$ in coupling reactions at various trypsin concentrations. Yields of HI-OMe (α) account for difference to 100%

Trypsin concentration T (mM) Time	Residual DAI, $100 - \alpha$			
	0.1	0.05	0.025	0.0125
1 min	89.2	91.3	97.4	98.7
2 min	78.4	84.9	92.8	97.0
4 min	60.0	73.7	87.9	93.9
6 min	47.4	65.2	81.9	91.6
8 min	37.6	57.7	77.5	86.0
10 min	30.5	50.4	71.9	85.9
15 min	17.7	35.6	63.0	77.4
30 min	5.7	15.5	40.4	60.9
45 min	4.1	9.3	24.7	46.9
1 h	4.2	6.9	20.4	36.1
4 h	3.2	5.1	5.2	6.9
k (min^{-1})	0.119	0.064	0.031	0.017
k/T (h^{-1} mM^{-1})	71	77	74	82
K_e(IM)	350	>210*	>210*	>150*

* Apparent decrease in K_e(IM) with decreasing concentrations of trypsin due to an increasing concentration of HI, accounted for as DAI, or by failing establishment of equilibrium

Conditions
Organic solvent	DMAC
H$_2$O, % nominal	20.7
Buffer (M/M)	HOAc/OAc$^-$ 1.5/1
Threonine ester	1 M Thr-OMe
Temperature (°C)	12
Calcium	3 mM
Substrate	8 mM DAI
Enzyme	Variable: 0.1, 0.05, 0.025, 0.0125 mM porcine trypsin TC

Analysis
Sampling (min)	1, 2, 4, 6, 8, 10, 15, 30, 45
(h)	1, 4
Preparation	NaCl/HCl precipitation
Method	HPLC, isocratic elution

Table 33 Yields of HI-OMe (α), DAI (β) and human insulin (γ) in transpeptidation reactions of human insulin to human insulin methyl ester

| | Insulin concentration (mM) | | | | | | | | | |
| | 2 | | | 4 | | | 8 | | | |
Time (h)	α	β(+γ)*	γ	α	β(+γ)*	γ	α	β(+γ)*	γ	Mean
0.17	4.2	95.8		4.8	95.2		2.9	97.1		
0.33	6.8	93.2		5.5	94.5		4.7	95.3		
0.5	8.9	91.1		7.4	92.6		7.1	92.9		
1	14.7	85.3		14.0	86.0		13.3	86.7		
2	26.3	73.3		26.1	73.9		25.0	75.0		
2.83	33.2	66.8		33.9	66.1		33.2	66.8		
4	43.3	56.7		42.4	57.6		44.6	55.4		
24	92.1	7.9		91.9	8.1		90.5	9.5		
48	89.3	10.7		90.6	9.4		—	—		
72	96.3	3.7		96.9	3.1		96.7	3.3		
144†	92.81	2.20	4.98	92.82	2.86	4.32	96.0	2.45	1.54	
k_{cat} (HI → IM) (h^{-1})		0.142			0.142			0.142		0.142
k_{cat} (HI → IM)/T (h^{-1} mM^{-1})										0.71
K_e(IM)		480			375			450		

*In samples up to 72 h DAI and HI were not chromatographically separated

Conditions
Organic solvent	DMAC
H$_2$O, % nominal	20.7
Buffer (M/M)	HOAc/OAc$^-$ 1.5/1
Threonine ester	1 M Thr-OMe
Temperature (°C)	12
Calcium	3 mM
Substrate	2, 4, 8 mM human insulin MC
Enzyme	0.2 mM porcine trypsin TC

Analysis
Sampling (h)	0.17, 0.33, 0.5, 1, 2, 2.83, 4, 24, 72, 144
Preparation	NaCl/HCl precipitation
Method	HPLC, gradient elution. Nucleosil 5 C$_{18}$ column
	† HPLC, isocratic elution Lichrosorb C$_{18}$ column (only 144 h samples)

Table 34 Yields of HI-OMe (α) and DOI plus DOI-Thr-OMe (β) in transpeptidation reactions. The specificity q and equilibrium constants K_e have been calculated for the varying concentrations of water and Thr-OMe, assuming equilibrium has been established after transpeptidation.

$K_e(\text{IM}) = [\text{HI-OMe}] \times [\text{H}_2\text{O}]/([\text{DAI}] \times [\text{Thr-OMe}])$

$[\text{H}_2\text{O}] = 0.555 \times \text{H}_2\text{O}\%$

Thr-OMe (M)	1	0.5	0.25	0.125	0.063
H$_2$O (%)	17.6	25.1	28.8	31.0	31.7
HI-OMe (α) (%)	93	89	76	54	43
DAI* $(1 - \alpha - \beta)$(%)	7†	4	7	11	16
DOI + DOI-Thr-OMe (β) (%)	0	7	17	35	41
Specificity q	—	>19	>7	>2.3	>1.7
K_e(IM)	130†	600	700	700	750

* DAI includes unconverted PI and possibly HI from HI-OMe hydrolysis
† Incomplete transpeptidation, Thr-OMe inhibits the reaction

Conditions

Organic solvent	DMAC
H$_2$O, % nominal	17.6, 25.1, 28.8, 31.0, 31.7
Buffer (M/M)	HOAc/OAc⁻ in constant ratio of 1.5/1: 1.5/1, 0.75/0.5, 0.37/0.25, 0.187/0.125, 0.094/0.063
Threonine ester	1, 0.5, 0.25, 0.125, 0.063 M Thr-OMe
Temperature (°C)	12
Calcium	3 mM
Substrate	8 mM porcine insulin FC
Enzyme	0.2 mM porcine trypsin TC

Analysis

Sampling (h)	24
Preparation	Acetone precipitation
Method	HPLC, isocratic elution

Table 35 Residual porcine insulin $(100 - \alpha)$ in transpeptidation reactions at various concentrations of Thr-OMe. Yields of HI-OMe (α) account for the difference to 100%

Time (h)	Threonine ester	
	1 M Thr-OMe	0.1 M Thr-OMe + 0.9 M NMM
	$100 - \alpha$	$100 - \alpha$
0.17	95.9	94.3
0.33	92.6	88.6
0.5	90.1	82.9
0.67	86.5	78.6
0.83	83.7	74.0
1	82.3	70.6
2	66.6	54.6
3	55.0	44.8
4	44.5	34.4
5	38.4	30.4
24	4.1	17.3
K(IM)	$> 270*$	550
k(h^{-1})	0.19	0.35
k/T(h^{-1} mM^{-1})	0.95	1.75

*Formation of HI from hydrolysis of HI-OMe accounted for as DAI and equilibrium not established in 1 M Thr-OMe

Conditions
Organic solvent   DMAC
H_2O, % nominal 20.7
Buffer (M/M)   HOAc/OAc$^-$ 1.5/1
Threonine ester   1 M Thr-OMe and 0.1 M Thr-OMe plus 0.9 M N-methyl morpholine (NMM)
Temperature (°C)   12
Calcium   3 mM
Substrate   8 mM porcine insulin MC
Enzyme   0.2 mM porcine trypsin TC

Analysis
Sampling (h)   0.17, 0.33, 0.5, 0.67, 0.83, 1, 2, 3, 4, 5, 24
Preparation   NaCl/HCl precipitation
Method   HPLC, isocratic elution

Table 36 Residual DAI $(100 - \alpha)$ in coupling reactions at various trypsin concentrations. Yields of HI(Bu^t)-OBu^t (α) account for the difference to 100%

Trypsin concentration, T(mM) Time	Residual DAI, $100 - \alpha$			
	0.1	0.05	0.025	0.0125
1 min	93.4	96.7	98.4	99.2
2 min	90.1	94.4	97.1	98.7
4 min	81.1	90.7	94.3	97.6
6 min	76.6	86.5	92.5	96.6
8 min	68.8	82.7	90.8	95.7
10 min	63.3	79.0	88.0	94.6
15 min	49.0	70.1	82.1	92.1
30 min	22.0	48.2	68.7	85.6
45 min	11.4	32.8	58.8	79.1
1 h	5.9	22.2	46.5	76.1
4 h	2.6	2.8	5.5	30.6
k(min^{-1})	0.051	0.022	0.013	0.005
k/T(min^{-1}mM^{-1})	0.51	0.44	0.52	0.40
K_e(IB)	430	400	>200*	>25*

* Reactions not yet settled at equilibrium cause an apparent decrease in K_e(IB) with decreasing trypsin concentration

Conditions
Organic solvent	DMAC
H$_2$O, % nominal	20.7
Buffer (M/M)	HOAc/OAc$^-$ 1.5/1
Threonine ester	1 M Thr(Bu^t)-OBu^t
Temperature (°C)	12
Calcium	3 mM
Substrate	8 mM DAI
Enzyme	Variable: 0.1, 0.05, 0.025, 0.0125 mM porcine trypsin TC

Analysis
Sampling (min)	1, 2, 4, 6, 8, 10, 15, 30, 45
(h)	1, 4
Preparation	NaCl/HCl precipitation
Method	HPLC, gradient elution

Table 37 Rate constants and equilibrium constants for coupling (DAI) and transpeptidation (porcine insulin) reactions in Thr(Bu^t)-OBu^t

	Coupling				
Substrate: DAI (mM)	8	6	4	2	Mean ± SD
k (min^{-1})	0.144	0.134	0.141	0.155	
k/T (min^{-1} mM^{-1})	0.720	0.670	0.705	0.775	0.72 ± 0.04
K_e(IB)*	350	300	230	—	300 ± 60
	Transpeptidation				
Substrate: porcine insulin (mM)	8	6	4	2	
k (min^{-1})	0.0079	0.0082	0.0074	0.0091	
k/T (min^{-1} mM^{-1})	0.0395	0.0410	0.0369	0.0456	0.041 ± 0.004
K_e(IB)†	335	350	270	250	300 ± 50
H$_2$O, K. F. analysis, % (w/v)	20.20	20.60	20.59	20.88	20.6 ± 0.3

* 60 min
† 1440 min

Conditions
Organic solvent   DMAC
H$_2$O, % nominal Coupling 22.0, transpeptidation 20.7
Buffer (M/M)   HOAc/OAc$^-$ 1.5/1
Threonine ester   1 M Thr(Bu^t)-OBu^t
Temperature (°C)   12
Calcium   3 mM
Substrate   8, 6, 4, 2 mM DAI; 8, 6, 4, 2 mM porcine insulin MC
Enzyme   0.2 mM; porcine trypsin TC

Analysis
Sampling (min)   Coupling: 1, 2, 3, 4, 5, 7, 10, 15, 20, 30, 40, 60
                   Transpeptidation: 5, 10, 15, 30, 60, 120, 1440
Preparation   Acetone precipitation
Method   HPLC, gradient elution

TABLES

Table 38 Yields of HI-OMe (α_1) and HI(Bu^t)-OBu^t (α_2) in % in transpeptidation reactions. The difference to 100% is unconverted porcine insulin and DAI

	Insulin concentration (mM)							
	2		4		8		16	
Time (h)	α_1	α_2	α_1	α_2	α_1	α_2	α_1	α_2
0.25	8.7	0.7	9.1	0.8	9.5	0.8	—	—
0.5	12.1	1.3	13.1	1.3	14.3	1.4	—	—
1	25.0	5.0	24.0	3.6	26.4	5.3	—	—
2	32.9	8.8	31.7	8.1	34.7	7.8	33.8	10.3
4	42.1	16.9	41.5	15.1	44.4	18.6	43.2	17.1
24	59.1	30.9	53.9	42.1	54.4	40.8	54.1	41.2
48	53.3	41.1	55.2	39.2	54.4	39.7	53.4	39.1
72	53.1	43.5	53.6	42.8	52.3	44.0	52.8	43.5
k(IA → IM)* (h^{-1})	0.31		0.32		0.35		—	
k(IA → IB)(h^{-1})	0.030		0.033		0.034		—	
k(IA → IM)/k(IA → IB)	10		10		10		—	
K_e(IM)/K_e(IB)†	1.22		1.25		1.19		1.21	

* Estimates derived from initial observations
† Calculated from data at 72 h

Conditions
Organic solvent   DMAC
H$_2$O, % nominal 22.0
Buffer (M/M)   HOAc/OAc$^-$ 1.5/1
Threonine ester   0.5 M Thr-OMe + 0.5 M Thr(Bu^t)-OBu^t
Temperature (°C) 12
Calcium   2 mM
Substrate   4, 8, 12, 16 mM porcine insulin MC
Enzyme   0.2 mM porcine trypsin TC

Analysis
Sampling (h)   0.25, 0.5, 1, 2, 4, 24, 48, 72
Preparation   NaCl/HCl precipitations
Method   HPLC, gradient elution

Table 39 Coupling of DAI to Thr-OMe (α_1) or Thr(Bu^t)-Bu^t (α_2), separately and mixed in a molar ratio of 1/1. Yields in %, the difference to 100% is DAI

Time (h)	1 M Thr-OMe	1 M Thr(Bu^t)-OBu^t	0.5 M Thr-OMe + 0.5 M Thr(Bu^t)-OBu^t	
	α_1	α_2	α_1	α_2
0.25	89.0	77.9	—	—
0.5	90.9	91.1	77.7	13.9
1	93.2	94.7	74.5	17.9
4	95.2	94.1	62.1	32.7
24	96.3	95.8	51.9	43.7
K_e(IM)*	299			
K_e(IB)*		262		
K_e(IM)/K_e(IB)			1.19	

* K_e calculation from equilibrium data at 24 h

Conditions
Organic solvent   DMAC
H$_2$O, % nominal   20.7
Buffer (M/M)   HOAc/OAc$^-$ 1.5/1
Threonine ester   1 M Thr-OMe and 1 M Thr(Bu^t)-OBu^t, and 0.5 M Thr-OMe plus 0.5 M Thr (Bu^t)-OBu^t mixed
Temperature (°C)   12
Calcium   3 mM
Substrate   8 mM DAI
Enzyme   0.2 mM porcine trypsin TC

Analysis
Sampling (h)   0.25, 0.5, 1, 2, 4, 24
Preparation   Acetone precipitation
Method   HPLC, gradient elution

Table 40 Yields of HI-OMe (α) and DOI plus DOI-Thr-OMe (β) in coupling reactions at 30 and 37°C. Yields in %

	H^+-Thr-OMe/H-Thr-OMe (M/M)							
	0.8/0.8				0/1.6			
Temp (°C)	30		37		30		37	
Time (h)	α	β	α	β	α	β	α	β
1	89	0	55	0	74	9	73	1
2	90	0	55	0	74	9	63	1
4	94	0	55	0	76	11	58	1
24	92	0	54	0	72	13	58	1
K_e(IM)	>110*		*		>30*		>20†	

* Enzyme inactivation before establishment of equilibrium
† Rapid hydrolysis of HI-OMe into HI at 37°C results in underestimated K_e(IM) values

Conditions

Organic solvent	DMAC
H_2O, % nominal	20.0
Buffer (M/M)	H^+-Thr-OMe/H-Thr-OMe 0/1.6, 0.8/0.8
Threonine ester	1.6 M Thr-OMe
Temperature (°C)	30, 37
Calcium	8 mM
Substrate	3.8% (w/v) DAI
Enzyme	0.38% (w/v) porcine trypsin TC

Analysis

Sampling (h)	1, 2, 4, 24
Preparation	NaCl/HCl precipitation
Method	HPLC, isocratic elution

Table 41 Yields of HI-OR (α), DAI (α_1), DOI plus DOI-Thr-OR (β) in transpeptidation reactions of SCI. The difference to 100% is accounted for by unconverted SCI

	Yields (%)			
Threonine ester	α	α_1	β	K_e
Thr(Bu^t)-OBu^t	74	2	3	430 K_e(IB)
Thr-OBu^t	48	5	2	110 K_e(ISB)
Thr-OTmb	63	3	5	240 K_e(ITmb)*

* Thr-OTmb not completely dissolved in reaction medium

Conditions

Organic solvent	DMAC
H_2O, % nominal	20.9
Buffer (M/M)	HOAc/OAc$^-$ 1.5/1
Threonine ester	1 M Thr(Bu^t)-OBu^t, 1 M Thr-OBu^t, 1 M Thr-OTmb (suspension)
Temperature (°C)	12
Calcium	5 mM
Substrate	5% (w/v) SCI(ge)
Enzyme	0.5% (w/v) porcine trypsin TC

Analysis

Sampling (h)	72
Preparation	Acetone precipitation
Method	HPLC, gradient elution

Table 42 Yields of HI(Bu^t)-OBu^t (α), DAI (α_1), DOI (β_1) and DOI-Thr(Bu^t)-OBu^t (β_2) in transpeptidation reactions of SCI. The difference to 100% is unconverted SCI. The late appearance of DOI and DOI-Thr(Bu^t)-OBu^t points towards an increased susceptibility of the Arg^{B22}-Gly^{B23} bond after cleavage of the Lys^{B29}-Gly^{A1} bond

BD/DMAC (v/v)	1/4								1/1								4/1							
Temp. (°C)	25				12				25				12				25				12			
Time (h)	α	α_1	β_2	β_1	α	α_1	β_2	β_1	α	α_1	β_2	β_1	α	α_1	β_2	β_1	α	α_1	β_2	β_1	α	α_1	β_2	β_1
4	25	0	0	0	6	0	0	0	29	0	0	0	8	0	0	0	25	5	1	0	7	2	0	0
22	50	4	0	0	28	5	0	0	55	4	1	6	34	3	0	0	48	5	2	12	35	4	0	3
48	61	2	0	0	54	3	0	0	58	4	3	9	56	4	2	4	—	—	—	—	48	5	2	8
73	—	—	—	—	58	3	1	0	56	3	4	8	60	4	3	6	45	4	12	17	52	5	5	10
K_e(IB)*	270				170				150				130				90				90			
K_e(DB)	—				—				4				4				6				4			

* Equilibrium constant determined using last observation

Conditions
Organic solvent	BD/DMAC 1/4, 1/1, 4/1 (v/v)
H$_2$O, % nominal	20.0
Buffer (M/M)	HOAc/OAc$^-$ 1.80/1.25
Threonine ester	1.25 M Thr(Bu^t)-OBu^t
Temperature (°C)	12, 25
Calcium	6 mM
Substrate	0.5% (w/v) SCI(ss)
Enzyme	0.1% (w/v) porcine trypsin TC

Analysis
Sampling (h)	4, 22, 48, 73
Preparation	Acetone precipitation
Method	HPLC, gradient elution

Table 43 Yields in % of HI-OR (α), DAI (α_1) and DOI plus DOI-Thr-OR (β) in transpeptidations of SCI in two threonine esters and in two solvents. The difference to 100% is accounted for by unconverted SCI

Solvent	Thr-OMe						Thr(Bu^t)-OBu^t					
	DMSO/BD			DMAC			DMSO/BD			DMAC		
Time (h)	α	α_1	β	α	α_1	β	α	α_1	β	α	α_1	β
24	11	0	0	5	0	0	4	0	0	31	1	2
48	21	0	0	9	0	0	7	0	4	55	1	4
72	30	2	1	12	0	0	11	0	5	69	1	3
144	42	3	2	16	0	0	18	4	4	82	2	5
216	46	3	2	18	0	1	26	3	8	—	—	—
K_e(IM)	170			—								
K_e(IB)							100			450		
k(h^{-1})	0.005			0.002			0.0015			0.016		

Conditions
Organic solvent	DMAC, DMSO/BD 1/1 (v/v)
H_2O, % nominal	19.8
Buffer (M/M)	HOAc/OAc$^-$ 1.5/1
Threonine ester	1 M Thr-OMe, 1 M Thr(Bu^t)-OBu^t
Temperature (°C)	12
Calcium	4 mM
Substrate	5% (w/v) SCI(ss)
Enzyme	0.4% (w/v) porcine trypsin TC

Analysis
Sampling (h)	24, 48, 72, 144, 216
Preparation	Acetone precipitation
Method	HPLC, gradient elution

Table 44 Yields of HI-OMe (α), DAI (α_1), and DOI plus DOI-Thr-OMe (β) in transpeptidation reactions of SCI in various solvents. The difference to 100% is accounted for by unconverted SCI

Solvent	DMSO						DMSO/BD* 4/1 (v/v)						DMSO/BD 1/1 (v/v)					
Temp. (°C)	12			25			12			25			12			25		
Time (h)	α	α_1	β	α	α_1	β	α	α_1	β	α	α_1	β	α	α_1	β	α	α_1	β
1.5	2	0	0	3	0	0	3	0	0	2	0	0	4	0	0	2	0	0
4	2	0	0	2	0	0	8	0	0	5	0	0	6	0	0	23	2	2
24	—	—	—	—	—	—	22	0	0	7	0	0	31	3	3	49	3	4
48	—	—	—	—	—	—	32	1	0	6	0	0	47	3	5	51	2	3
118	—	—	—	—	—	—	42	0	0	5	0	0	49	7	11	49	2	3
K_e(IM)															100		300	

* Zero values for DAI due to low insulin concentrations caused by fibril formation

Conditions
Organic solvent   DMSO; DMSO/BD 4/1, 1/1 (v/v)
H_2O, % nominal   19.8
Buffer (M/M)   HOAc/OAc⁻ 1.5/1
Threonine ester   1 M Thr-OMe
Temperature (°C)   12, 25
Calcium   5 mM
Substrate   0.5% (w/v) SCI(ss)
Enzyme   0.5% (w/v) porcine trypsin TC

Analysis
Sampling (h)   1.5, 4, 24, 48, 118
Preparation   Acetone precipitation
Method   HPLC, isocratic elution

Table 45 Yields of HI-OBuᵗ (α), DAI (α_1), DOI (β_1), and DOI-Thr-OBuᵗ (β_2) in transpeptidation reactions of SCI

H₂O (%)	19.8															
Solvent	DMAC								DMAC/BD 8/2							
Temp. (°C)	12				20				12				20			
Time (h)	α	α_1	β_2	β_1	α	α_1	β_2	β_1	α	α_1	β_2	β_1	α	α_1	β_2	β_1
24	8	0	0	0	13	0	0	0	12	0	0	0	24	1	2	0
48	15	0	0	0	18	0	0	0	20	1	1	0	40	1	3	0
120	31	1	0	0	22	0	0	0	40	1	3	0	56	3	7	0
K_e(ISB)	340								440				200			

H₂O (%)	25.6															
Solvent	DMAC/BD 7/3								DMAC/BD 6/4							
Temp. (°C)	12				20				12				20			
Time (h)	α	α_1	β_2	β_1	α	α_1	β_2	β_1	α	α_1	β_2	β_1	α	α_1	β_2	β_1
24	36	5	5	2	51	8	15	5	33	6	7	3	48	5	17	5
48	49	11	7	5	49	5	30	11	44	6	18	8	49	5	28	10
120	47	10	40	9	24	63*		12	33	50*		14	25	59*		14
K_e(ISB)	70				140				100				140			
K_e(DSB)	60				40				30				40			

*DAI (α_1) contained in DOI-Thr-OBuᵗ (β_2) peak at higher concentrations of the latter

Conditions
Organic solvent   DMAC/BD 8/2, 7/3, 6/4; DMAC
H₂O, % nominal   19.8, 25.6
Buffer (M/M)   HOAc/OAc⁻ 1.5/1
Threonine ester   1 M Thr-OBuᵗ
Temperature (°C)   12, 20
Calcium   5 mM
Substrate   1.25% (w/v) SCI(ss)
Enzyme   0.5% (w/v) porcine trypsin TC

Analysis
Sampling (h)   24, 48, 120
Preparation   Acetone precipitation
Method   HPLC, gradient eluent

Table 46 Activation energies in coupling and transpeptidation reactions in DMAC. Arrhenius plots are nonlinear, reaction rates drop more than expected from 277 to 273°K for both reactions

Trypsin (mM)	Temp. (°K)	Coupling, k (min^{-1})			E_A (kJ/mole)
		273	277	285	
0.2			0.083	0.157	52
0.02			0.0093	0.0166	48
0.02		0.0041	0.0093		129

Trypsin (mM)	Temp. (°K)	Transpeptidation, k (h^{-1})			E_A (kJ/mole)
		273	277	285	
0.2		0.0415		0.184	80
			0.091	0.170	51
			0.078	0.178	68
		0.0415	0.078		99

Conditions

Organic solvent	DMAC
H_2O, % nominal	20.7
Buffer (M/M)	HOAc/OAc$^-$ 1.5/1
Threonine ester	1 M Thr-OMe
Temperature (°K)	273, 277, 285
Calcium	5 mM
Substrate	8 mM DAI and porcine insulin MC
Enzyme	0.2 mM and 0.02 mM porcine trypsin TC

Analysis

Sampling (h)	0.17, 0.33, 0.5, 0.67, 0.83, 1, 1.5, 2, 3, 4 (transpeptidation)
(min)	1, 2, 3, 4, 5, 6, 8, 10, 15, 30, 60 (coupling)
Preparation	NaCl/HCl precipitation
Method	HPLC, isocratic elution

Table 47 Yields of HI-OMe (α) in % in coupling reactions. In the highly acidic buffers using HOAc/OAc⁻ ratios of 9/1 and 19/1 the reaction is virtually stopped, even at 26.9 and 34% water

	H^+-Thr-OMe/Thr-OMe (M/M)		HOAc/OAc⁻ (M/M)					
	0.5/0.5	0/1	1.5/1	4/1	6/0.67	7.6/0.4	6/0.67	7.6/0.4
H_2O (%)	18.4	17.5	20.7	20.0	20.2	20.7	26.9	34.0
Time (h)	α	α	α	α	α	α	α	α
1/2		85						
1	95	95	94	36	3	3	3	3
2	96	95	92	54	2	3	2	3
4	93	93	92	73	1	1	1	1
24	96	90	95	85	2	2	3	2

Conditions

Organic solvent	DMAC
H_2O, % nominal	Variable, from 17.5 to 34
Buffer (M/M)	HOAc/OAc⁻ 1.5/1, 4/1, 6/0.67, 7.6/0.4
	H^+-Thr-OMe/Thr-OMe 0/1, 0.5/0.5
Threonine ester	1 M, 0.67 M, 0.4 M Thr-OMe
Temperature (°C)	12
Calcium	3 mM
Substrate	5% (w/v) DAI
Enzyme	0.5% (w/v) porcine trypsin TC

Analysis

Sampling (h)	0.5, 1, 2, 4, 24
Preparation	Acetone precipitation
Method	HPLC, isocratic elution

Table 48 Yields of HI-OMe (α) and DOI plus DOI-Thr-OMe (β) in transpeptidation reactions in H^+-Thr-OMe/Thr-OMe buffers, in which the counter ion is either chloride or acetate

	H^+-Thr-OMe/Thr-OMe (M/M)									
	0/0.7		0.35/0.35				0.7/0			
Cl^- (M)	0		0.35		0		0.7		0	
OAc^- (M)	0		0		0.35		0		0.7	
H_2O (%)	29.2		28.1		27.1		25.1		25.1	
Yields	α	β	α	β	α	β	α	β	α	β
4 h	36	57	42	8	56	11	0	2	25	5
24 h	31	59	40	8	53	13	0	3	24	7

Conditions

Organic solvent	DMAC
H_2O, % nominal	Variable, range 25.1–29.2
Buffer (M/M)	H^+-Thr-OMe/Thr-OMe 0/0.7, 0.35/0.35, 0.7/0
Threonine ester	0.7 M Thr-OMe
Temperature (°C)	37
Calcium	2 mM
Chloride ions	0, 0.35, 0.7 M
Substrate	3.5% (w/v) porcine insulin FC
Enzyme	0.35% (w/v) porcine trypsin TC

Analysis

Sampling (h)	4, 24
Preparation	Acetone precipitation
Method	HPLC, isocratic elution

Table 49 Yields of HI-OMe estimated by visual observation of stained PAGE gels

	Buffer	Pyridinium, Cl^-	Pyridinium, OAc^-	HOAc	HOAc
	H_2O (%)	pyridine 35	pyridine 30	Na^+, OAc^- 43	K^+, OAc^- 43
Thr-OR	Solvent				
Thr-OMe	DMF	0	50	50	50
	DMSO	0	60	5*	40
	DMF	0	60	60	60
Thr-OBu^t	DMSO	0	60	20*	50*

* DOI is visible, see Figure 18

Conditions

Organic solvent	DMF, DMSO	
H_2O, % nominal	35, 30, 43	
Buffer (M/M)	Pyridinium chloride/pyridine	0.9/0.9
	Pyridinium acetate/pyridine	0.9/0.9
	HOAc/NaOAc	0.9/0.9
	HOAc/KOAc	0.9/0.9
Threonine ester	0.5 M Thr-OMe and 0.5 M Thr-OBu^t	
Temperature (°C)	37	
Calcium	0 mM	
Substrate	5% (w/v) DAI	
Enzyme	0.6% (w/v) TPCK treated trypsin	

Analysis

Sampling (h)	24
Preparation	10 × dilution in application buffer in 8 M urea
Method	Disc electrophoresis

Table 50 Yields of HI-OMe (α), DOI (β_1), and DOI-Thr-OMe (β_2) in buffers comprising formiate, acetate and phosphate counter ions

										Counter ion: $H_2PO_4^-$														
	Formic acid/formiate (M/M) 0.25/1						HOAc/OAc⁻ (M/M) 1.4/1						H⁺-Thr-OMe/Thr-OMe (M/M) 0.5/0.5						1/0					
H₂O (%)	34.5						27.8						33.9						33.6					
Temp. (°C)	12			21			12			21			12			21			12			21		
	α	β_1	β_2	α	β_1	β_2	α	β_1	β_2	α	β_1	β_2	α	β_1	β_2	α	β_1	β_2	α	β_1	β_2	α	β_1	β_2
4	0	0	0	0	0	0	8	0	0	6	0	0	55	3	20	37	5	45	0	0	0	0	0	0
24	0	0	0	0	0	0	20	1	1	6	0	0	26	5	67	6	8	85	0	0	0	0	0	0
48	0	0	0	0	0	0	22	1	1	8	0	0	4	7	87	1	10	88	0	0	0	0	0	0
Specificity q													5				2							

Conditions

Organic solvent	Acetamide
H₂O, % nominal	Variable, range 27.8–34.5
Buffer (M/M)	Formic acid/formiate 0.25/1; HOAc/OAc⁻ 1.4/1; H⁺-Thr-OMe/Thr-OMe 0.5/0.5, 1/0, counter ion H₂PO₄⁻
Threonine ester	1 M Thr-OMe
Temperature (°C)	12, 21
Calcium	3 mM
Substrate	6.7% (w/v) porcine insulin FC
Enzyme	0.67% (w/v) porcine trypsin TC

Analysis

Sampling (h)	4, 24, 48
Preparation	NaCl/HCl precipitation
Method	HPLC, isocratic elution

Table 51 Yields of HI-OMe (α) estimated by visual observation of stained PAGE gels

HOAc/OAc⁻ (M/M)	0/1	0.5/1	1/1	1.5/1
H₂O (%)	44.3	41.4	38.6	35.7
Substrate	α	α	α	α
Porcine insulin	10	50	20	5
DAI	15	70	70	50
Porcine proinsulin	30	60	50	40

Conditions

Organic solvent	DMF
H₂O, % nominal	35.7, 38.6, 41.4, 44.3
Buffer (M/M)	HOAc/OAc⁻ 0/1, 0.5/1, 1/1, 1.5/1
Threonine ester	1 M Thr-OMe
Temperature (°C)	37
Calcium	0 mM
Substrate	5% (w/v) DAI, porcine insulin MC, porcine proinsulin
Enzyme	0.6% (w/v) TPCK treated trypsin

Analysis

Sampling (h)	24
Preparation	10 × dilution in application buffer
Method	Disc electrophoresis

Table 52 Yields of HI-OMe (α) and DOI plus DOI-Thr-OMe (β) in transpeptidation reactions of various insulin compounds

Temp. (°C)	Arg^{B31}-Arg^{B32} porcine insulin				Mixture of des[Arg^{31}, Arg^{32}] porcine proinsulin and des[Lys^{62}, Arg^{63}] porcine proinsulin		Rabbit insulin (Ser^{B30} human insulin)	
	15		37		37		37	
	α	β	α	β	α	β	α	β
4 h	98	2	90	10	87	10	87	10
24 h	89	11	—	—	88	10	81	11

Conditions

Organic solvent	DMAC
H$_2$O, % nominal	31.4
Buffer (M/M)	HOAc/OAc$^-$ 0.5/1
Threonine ester	1 M Thr-OMe
Temperature (°C)	15, 37
Calcium	3 mM
Substrate	0.5% (w/v), various insulin compounds
Enzyme	0.3% (w/v) porcine trypsin TC

Analysis

Sampling (h)	4, 24
Preparation	Acetone precipitation
Method	HPLC, isocratic elution

Table 53 Yields of HI-OMe (α), DOI plus DOI-Thr-OMe (β), and specificity q in transpeptidation reactions using different trypsin preparations

EDTA (mM)	0						4.5					
Trypsin (%)	0.75			0.25			0.75			0.25		
Trypsin prep.	α	β	q	α	β	q	α	β	q	α	β	q
TPCK-treated (8/1-1980)	57	21	5	33	5	8	37	8	6	16	2	9
TPCK-treated (17/9-1979)	58	23	5	35	5	9	38	9	6	16	2	9
Once crystallized	49	44	4	54	13	7	39	10	5	16	2	9
Once crystallized, sterile	47	48	4	45	8	8	34	7	6	16	3	6
Twice crystallized	51	11	7	48	11	7	40	10	6	16	3	6

Conditions

Organic solvent	DMAC
H$_2$O, % nominal	41.4
Buffer (M/M)	HOAc/OAc$^-$ 0.5/1
Threonine ester	1 M Thr-OMe
Temperature (°C)	37
Calcium	0 mM
EDTA	0 and 4.5 mM
Substrate	5% (w/v) porcine insulin FC
Enzyme	0.25 and 0.75% (w/v) different preparations of trypsin, all porcine origin

Analysis

Sampling (h)	18
Preparation	Acetone precipitation
Method	HPLC, isocratic elution

Table 54 Yields of HI-OR estimated by visual observation of stained PAGE gels

Substrate	Thr-OR	Trypsin	Plasmin	Trypsin* imm. glass	Trypsin* imm. Sephadex
Porcine	Thr-OMe	90	0	80	30
insulin	Thr-OBu^t	40	0	2	30
Porcine	Thr-OMe	90	0	90	2
proinsulin	Thr-OBu^t	70	0	40	2

*Suspension of immobilized trypsin tended to form gels

Conditions

Organic solvent	DMAC
H$_2$O, % nominal	36.4 imm. enzymes, 41.4 soluble enzymes
Buffer (M/M)	HOAc/OAc$^-$ 0.5/1
Threonine ester	1 M Thr-OMe, 1 M Thr-OBu^t
Temperature (°C)	37
Calcium	0 mM
Substrate	5% (w/v) porcine insulin, porcine proinsulin
Enzyme	0.6% (w/v) TPCK treated trypsin
	0.6% (w/v) plasmin
	100 U/ml = 500 mg/ml immobilized trypsin, on glass beads
	150 U/ml = 100 mg/ml immobilized trypsin, on Sephadex G-150

Analysis

Sampling (h)	24
Preparation	10 × dilution in application buffer
Method	Disc electrophoresis

Table 55 Yields of HI-OMe using *Achromobacter lyticus* protease to catalyse transpeptidation reactions

Temperature (°C)	12			25					
H$_2$O (%)	27.7			23.2			27.7		
HOAc/OAc$^-$ (M/M)	1.2/1.2	0.6/1.2	0/1.2	1.2/1.2	0.6/1.2	0/1.2	1.2/1.2	0.6/1.2	0/1.2
Yields (%)	50	31	18	—	85	86	87	87	89

Conditions

Organic solvent	DMAC
H$_2$O, % nominal	23.2, 27.7
Buffer (M/M)	HOAc/OAc$^-$ 1.2/1.2, 0.6/1.2, 0/1.2
Threonine ester	1.2 M Thr-OMe
Temperature (°C)	12, 25
Calcium	6 mM
Substrate	6% (w/v) porcine insulin FC
Enzyme	2.4 AU/ml $\simeq$ 0.18% (w/v) *Achromobacter lyticus* protease (WAKO)

Analysis

Sampling (h)	72
Preparation	Acetone precipitation
Method	HPLC, isocratic elution

Table 56 Yields of HI-OMe in attempts to transpeptidize porcine insulin with various enzymes having specificity for basic amino acid residues

| | H^+-Thr-OMe/Thr-OMe (M/M) | | | |
| | 0.5/0.5 | | 1/0 | |
H_2O (%)	25.5	47.1	25.5	47.1
Streptokinase, 20 000 U/ml	0	0	0	0
Urokinase, 8250 U/ml	0	0	0	0
Enterokinase, 3.12 mg/ml	0	0	0	0

Conditions
Organic solvent   DMAC
H_2O, % nominal   25.5, 47.1
Buffer (M/M) H^+-Thr-OMe/Thr-OMe 0.5/0.5, 1/0
Threonine ester   1 M Thr-OMe
Temperature (°C)   37
Calcium   0 mM
Substrate   5% (w/v) porcine insulin FC
Enzyme   Streptokinase, urokinase and enterokinase

Analysis
Sampling (h)   24
Preparation   Acetone precipitation
Method   HPLC, isocratic elution

Table 57 Yields of DAI (α), DOI (β) and intermediate (γ) by cleaving SCI and SCI-AAK by trypsin activated plasmin (2 mg/ml) in a 0.05 M Tris buffer, pH 8.25, containing 0.01 M lysine and in a 0.05 M sodium acetate buffer, pH 5.5, containing 0.01 M lysine. Temperature 37°C. The difference in yields to 100% is accounted for by unconverted SCI or SCI-AAK

| | SCI, 5 mg/ml | | | | SCI-AAK, 10 mg/ml | | | | | |
| | 0.05 M Tris pH 8.25 | | 0.05 M acetate pH 5.5 | | 0.05 M Tris pH 8.25 | | | 0.05 M acetate pH 5.5 | | |
Time (h)	α	β	α	β	α	β	γ	α	β	γ
24	52	3	13	3	93	4	0	83	5	5
48	66	6	20	7	89	7	0	88	12	0
72	72	8	26	12	87	9	0	80	20	0

Table 58 Yield of HI-OR (α), DAI (α_1) and DOI plus DOI-Thr-OR (β) in transpeptidation reactions. The difference to 100% is unconverted SCI

Solvent % H₂O	DMSO/BD 1/1 19.7						DMAC 19.7						DMAC 20.7					
HOAc/OAc⁻ (M/M)	1.5/1						1.5/1						0/1					
Thr-OR	Thr-OMe			Thr(Buᵗ)-OBuᵗ			Thr-OMe			Thr(Buᵗ)-OBuᵗ			Thr-OMe			Thr(Buᵗ)-OBuᵗ		
Time, (h)	α	α_1	β	α	α_1	β	α	α_1	β	α	α_1	β	α	α_1	β	α	α_1	β
24	35	0	2	4	2	36	0	0	0	77	5	0	24	0	0	0	0	44
48	50	0	4	0	0	51	0	0	0	84	3	3	33	0	0	0	0	58
72	56	0	2	0	0	62	—	—	—	86	4	4	42	0	0	0	0	74
96	—	—	—	0	0	65	—	—	—	89	5	5	—	—	—	0	0	75
k(h⁻¹)	0.02			—			—			0.07			0.011			—		

Conditions

Organic solvent	DMAC, DMSO/BD 1/1
H₂O, % nominal	19.7, 20.7
Buffer (M/M)	HOAc/OAc⁻ 0/1, 1.5/1
Threonine ester	1 M Thr-OMe, 1 M Thr(Buᵗ)-OBuᵗ
Temperature (°C)	12
Calcium	4 mM
Substrate	0.5% (w/v) SCI (ss + ge)
Enzyme	0.5% (w/v) porcine trypsin TC

Analysis

Sampling (h)	24, 48, 72, 96
Preparation	Acetone precipitation
Method	HPLC, gradient elution

Table 59 Yields of HI-OBu^t (α), DOI (β_1) and DAI plus DOI-Thr-OBu^t ($\alpha_1\beta_2$) in transpeptidation reactions. The difference to 100% is unconverted SCI

Time (h)	DMF			Acetone			DMSO			DMAC		
	α	$\alpha_1\beta_2$	β_1	α	$\alpha_1\beta_2$	β_1	α	$\alpha_1\beta_2$	β_1	α	$\alpha_1\beta_2$	β_1
4.5	67	16	0	38	51	10	47	*	0	21	*	0
24	41	46	1	13	66	20	—	—	—	—	—	—
48	36	60	1	9	79	12	78	22	0	75	15	0
$k(\mathrm{h}^{-1})$	>0.25						>0.14			0.05		

* Peak not integrated

Conditions

Organic solvent	DMF, acetone, DMSO, DMAC, all mixed with BD 9/1 (v/v)
H$_2$O, % nominal	22.3
Buffer (M/M)	HOAc/OAc$^-$ 0/1.14
Threonine ester	1.14 M Thr-OBu^t
Temperature (°C)	12
Calcium	7 mM
Substrate	0.6% (w/v) SCI (ss)
Enzyme	0.7% (w/v) porcine trypsin TC

Analysis

Sampling (h)	4.5, 24, 48
Preparation	Acetone precipitation
Method	HPLC, gradient elution

Table 60 Yields of HI-OBu^t (α), DAI (α_1), DOI (β_1), and DOI-Thr-OBu^t (β_2) in transpeptidation reactions in various organic solvents, all mixed with BD in a ratio of 4.3/1. The difference to 100% is unconverted SCI

Time (h)	DMF				Acetone				DMSO				DMAC				t-Butanol			
	α	α_1	β_2	β_1	α	α_1	β_2	β_1	α	α_1	β_2	β_1	α	α_1	β_2	β_1	α	α_1	β_2	β_1
5	49	8	5	0	43	39*		13	32	5*		0	14	4*		0	42	42*		16
24	64	31*		3	10	72*		18	66	3	18	0	41	2	12	0	6	3	70	21
48	51	44*		5	0	81*		19	77	13	10	0	64	15*		0	0	0	77	23
72	35	54*		10	0	75*		25	68	27*		5	76	19*		4	0	0	72	28
144	12	70*		18	0	26*		74	53	36*		10	64	28*		8	0	0	71	29
$k(\mathrm{h}^{-1})$	0.18				—				0.08				0.03				—			

* DAI and DOI-Thr-OBu^t are not separated in the HPLC analysis

Conditions

Organic solvent	DMF, acetone, DMSO, DMAC, t-butanol, all mixed with BD 4.3/1 (v/v)
H$_2$O, % nominal	20.0
Buffer (M/M)	HOAc/OAc$^-$ 1.70/1.14
Threonine ester	1.14 M Thr-OBu^t
Temperature (°C)	12
Calcium	7 mM
Substrate	1.25% (w/v) SCI (ge)
Enzyme	0.7% (w/v) porcine trypsin TC

Analysis

Sampling (h)	5, 24, 48, 72, 144
Preparation	Acetone precipitation
Method	HPLC, gradient elution

Table 61   Yields of HI-OBuᵗ (α), DOI (β₁), and DAI plus DOI-Thr-OBuᵗ (α₁β₂). The difference to 100% is unconverted SCI. DAI and DOI-Thr-OBuᵗ coelute

DMAC/BD	0.5% trypsin (w/v)												1% trypsin (w/v)					
	1/0			11/1			1/1			0.85/1			1/0			11/1		
Time (h)	α	α₁β₂	β₁	α	α₁β₂	β₁	α	α₁β₂	β₁	α	α₁β₂	β₁	α	α₁β₂	β₁	α	α₁β₂	β₁
24	30	10	6	30	15	8	36	17	19	30	19	22	35	16	17	29	22	17
72	54	13	7	55	17	12	33	25	29	31	28	35	48	21	22	48	21	24
$k(h^{-1})$	>0.015			>0.015			>0.018			>0.015			>0.018			>0.014		

Conditions

Organic solvent	DMAC/BD 1/0, 11/1, 1/1, 0.85/1 (v/v)
H_2O, % nominal	20.7
Buffer (M/M)	HOAc/OAc⁻ 1.5/1
Threonine ester	1 M Thr-OBuᵗ
Temperature (°C)	12
Calcium	5 mM
Substrate	0.5% (w/v) SCI (ge)
Enzyme	0.5% and 1% (w/v) porcine trypsin TC

Analysis

Sampling (h)	24, 72
Preparation	Acetone precipitation
Method	HPLC, gradient elution

Table 62   Yields of HI-OBuᵗ (α), DAI (α₁), DOI (β₁), and DOI-Thr-OBuᵗ (β₂) in transpeptidation reactions. The difference to 100% is accounted for by unconverted SCI

DMAC/BD (v/v)	0/1				1/9				1/4				1/2			
Time (h)	α	α₁	β₂	β₁	α	α₁	β₂	β₁	α	α₁	β₂	β₁	α	α₁	β₂	β₁
24	20	3	6	0	19	3	6	0	18	2	3	0	10	0	0	0
48	26	5	15	3	24	6	15	3	27	5	8	2	14	1	3	0
96	28	36*		8	28	40*		10	34	29*		6	29	3	8	2
$k(h^{-1})$	0.01				0.01				0.01				0.004			

* DAI and DOI-Thr-OBuᵗ coelute

Conditions

Organic solvent	DMAC/BD 0/1, 1/9, 1/4, 1/2 (v/v)
H_2O, % nominal	12.5
Buffer (M/M)	HOAc/OAc⁻ 1.8/1.2
Threonine ester	1.2 M Thr-OBuᵗ
Temperature (°C)	12
Calcium	5 mM
Substrate	0.6% (w/v) SCI (ss)
Enzyme	0.6% (w/v) porcine trypsin TC

Analysis

Sampling (h)	24, 48, 96
Preparation	Acetone precipitation
Method	HPLC, gradient elution

Table 63 Yields of HI-OBu^t (α), DAI (α_1), DOI (β_1), and DOI-Thr-OBu^t (β_2) in transpeptidation reactions. The difference to 100% is accounted for by unconverted SCI

DMAC/BD (v/v)																
	5/5								4/6							
HOAc/OAc⁻ (M/M)	2/1				1.5/1				2/1				1.5/1			
H₂O (%)	22.6				25.5				22.6				25.5			
Time (h)	α	α_1	β_2	β_1	α	α_1	β_2	β_1	α	α_1	β_2	β_1	α	α_1	β_2	β_1
6	18	5	4	2	25	4	5	1	16	1	1	0	24	5	5	0
24	32	8	21	7	42	11	20	5	38	4	12	1	35	10	24	6
48	31	5	39	11	34	7	44	8	42	6	27	4	26	5	49	12
k(h⁻¹)	0.05				0.06				0.03				0.06			

Conditions

Organic solvent	DMAC/BD 5/5, 4/6 (v/v)
H₂O, % nominal	22.6, 25.5
Buffer (M/M)	HOAc/OAc⁻ 1.5/1, 2/1
Threonine ester	1 M Thr-OBu^t
Temperature (°C)	18
Calcium	5 mM
Substrate	1.25% (w/v) SCI (ss)
Enzyme	0.5% (w/v) porcine trypsin TC

Analysis

Sampling; (h)	6, 24, 48
Preparation	Acetone precipitation
Method	HPLC, gradient elution

Table 64 Yields of HI-OMe (α), DAI (α_1) and DOI plus DOI-Thr-OMe (β) in transpeptidation reactions of SCI. The difference to 100% is unconverted SCI

DMSO/BD	4/6						3/7						2/8					
Temp. (°C)	12			25			12			25			12			25		
Time (h)	α	α_1	β	α	α_1	β	α	α_1	β	α	α_1	β	α	α_1	β	α	α_1	β
24	12	5	1	33	6	34	11	8	2	29	4	45	10	5	.	22	3	56
48	24	4	3	34	5	49	22	5	22	25	*	74	20	*	27	13	*	87
72	29	6	22	30	7	55	25	6	30	19	3	78	—	—	—	—	—	—
k(h⁻¹)	0.008			0.04			0.009			0.04			0.007			0.04		

* Peak is not integrated

Conditions

Organic solvent	DMSO/BD 4/6, 3/7, 2/8 (v/v)
H₂O, % nominal	19.75
Buffer (M/M)	HOAc/OAc⁻ 1.5/1
Threonine ester	1 M Thr-OBu^t
Temperature (°C)	12, 25
Calcium	4 mM
Substrate	0.5% (w/v) SCI (ss)
Enzyme	0.5% (w/v) porcine trypsin TC

Analysis

Sampling (h)	24, 48, 72
Preparation	Acetone precipitation
Method	HPLC, isocratic elution

158

Table 65 Yields of HI-OBu^t (α), DAI (α_1), DOI (β_1) and DOI-Thr-OBu^t (β_2) in transpeptidation reactions. DOI-Thr-OBu^t and DAI are not resolved by HPLC analysis. Difference between H$_2$O% Karl Fischer (K.F.) and H$_2$O% nominal amounts to 1.1% on average

HOAc/OAc⁻ (M/M)									0.28/1.14			0.57/1.14			1.14/1.14		
H$_2$O%, K.F.	22.53			22.59			21.14			20.73			21.91			22.47		
Time (h)	α	$\alpha_1\beta_2$	β_1	α	$\alpha_1\beta_2$	β_1	α	$\alpha_1\beta_2$	β_1	α	$\alpha_1\beta_2$	β_1	α	$\alpha_1\beta_2$	β_1	α	$\alpha_1\beta_2$	β_1
24	84	15	1	90	9	1	84	12	1	75	7	0	75	5	0	66	7	0
48	76	22	2	81	17	2	83	9	1	83	9	0	82	12	0	77	13	0
72	72	22	7	76	24	0	72	24	4	81	13	3	81	16	2	76	18	2

Conditions

Organic solvent	DMF
H$_2$O, % nominal	21.0
Buffer (M/M)	HOAc/OAc⁻ 0/1.14, 0.28/1.14, 0.57/1.14, 1.14/1.14
Threonine ester	1.14 M Thr-OBu^t
Temperature (°C)	12
Calcium	7 mM
Substrate	5.7% (w/v) SCI (ge)
Enzyme	0.6% (w/v) porcine trypsin TC

Analysis

Sampling (h)	24, 48, 72
Preparation	Acetone precipitation
Method	HPLC, gradient elution

Table 66 Yields of HI-OBu^t (α), DAI (α_1), DOI (β_1) and DOI-Thr-OBu^t (β_2) in transpeptidation reactions. DOI-Thr-OBu^t and DAI are not resolved by HPLC analysis. Difference between H$_2$O% Karl Fischer (K.F.) and H$_2$O% nominal amounts to 1.7% on average

	$HOAc/OAc^-$ 0.28/1.14								
H$_2$O%, nominal	19.0			20.0			21.0		
H$_2$O% K.F. analysis	19.9			22.37			22.57		
Time (h)	α	$\alpha_1\beta_2$	β_1	α	$\alpha_1\beta_2$	β_1	α	$\alpha_1\beta_2$	β_1
24	27	7	0	48	12	2	50	12	2
48	39	7	0	71	14	1	72	15	1
72	44	7	0	75	17	1	76	18	1
144	50	8	0	74	26	0	71	26	2

	$HOAc/OAc^-$ 0.14/1.14								
H$_2$O%, nominal	19.0			20.0			21.0		
H$_2$O% K.F. analysis	20.15			21.62			23.21		
Time (h)	α	$\alpha_1\beta_2$	β_1	α	$\alpha_1\beta_2$	β_1	α	$\alpha_1\beta_2$	β_1
24	34	9	1	45	10	1	56	13	2
48	51	9	0	68	12	0	75	8	1
72	57	9	0	74	14	0	75	22	1
144	63	11	0	78	19	0	66	32	2

	$HOAc/OAc^-$ 0/1.14					
H$_2$O%, nominal	19.0			20.0		
H$_2$O% K.F. analysis	20.95			21.76		
Time (h)	α	$\alpha_1\beta_2$	β_1	α	$\alpha_1\beta_2$	β_1
24	43	10	1	56	12	1
48	62	11	0	73	14	2
72	67	12	0	77	17	1
144	75	14	0	76	23	0

Conditions
Organic solvent	DMF
H$_2$O, % nominal	19, 20, 21
Buffer (M/M)	HOAc/OAc$^-$ 0/1.14, 0.14/1.14, 0.28/1.14
Threonine ester	1.14 M Thr-OBu^t
Temperature (°C)	12
Calcium	7 mM
Substrate	5% (w/v) SCI (ge)
Enzyme	0.6% (w/v) porcine trypsin TC

Analysis
Sampling (h)	24, 48, 72, 144
Preparation	Acetone precipitation
Method	HPLC, gradient elution

Table 67 First order rate constants for formation of HI-OBu^t from SCI as a function of the concentration of water

H_2O (%)	0.24 mM trypsin				
	19*	18	17	16	15
$k(\mathrm{h}^{-1})$	0.108	0.059	0.029	0.014	0.0068
$k/T(\mathrm{h}^{-1}\,\mathrm{mM}^{-1})$	0.54	0.30	0.15	0.07	0.034

H_2O (%)	0.12 mM trypsin		
	19	18	17
$k\,(\mathrm{h}^{-1})$	0.046	0.035	0.018
$k/T\,(\mathrm{h}^{-1}\,\mathrm{mM}^{-1})$	0.38	0.29	0.15

*Formation of DOI-Thr-OMe plus DAI (unresolved peak) amounted to 18% after 72 h in 19% water in DMF. At lower water concentrations DOI formation was virtually suppressed.

Conditions
Organic solvent   DMF
H_2O, % nominal   15, 16, 17, 18, 19
Buffer (M/M)   HOAc/OAc$^-$ 0/1.14
Threonine ester   1.14 M Thr-OBu^t
Temperature (°C)   12
Calcium   7 mM
Substrate   1.25% (w/v) SCI (ss)
Enzyme   0.24 mM, 0.12 mM porcine trypsin TC

Analysis
Sampling (h)   6, 24, 48, 72
Preparation   Acetone precipitation
Method   HPLC, gradient elution

Table 68 Yields of HI-OBu^t (α), DAI (α_1), DOI (β_1) and DOI-Thr-OBu^t (β_2) in transpeptidation reactions using different concentrations of trypsin. DOI-Thr-OBu^t and DAI are not resolved by HPLC analysis

Trypsin (%)	0.28						0.43						Mean
H$_2$O (%) K.F.	21.60			21.23			21.65			21.33			21.45
Time (h)	α	$\alpha_1\beta_2$	β_1	α	$\alpha_1\beta_2$	β_1	α	$\alpha_1\beta_2$	β_1	α	$\alpha_1\beta_2$	β_1	
24	58	4	1	56	3	1	67	7	1	70	5	1	
48	79	8	0	77	7	0	82	11	1	83	9	0	
72	83	11	0	83	10	0	82	16	0	84	13	0	
96	84	13	0	85	11	0	79	20	0	83	16	0	
168	78	21	0	80	20	0	69	31	0	75	24	0	

Conditions
Organic solvent   DMF
H$_2$O, % nominal   21.0
Buffer (M/M)   HOAC/OAc$^-$ 0/1.14
Threonine ester   1.14 M Thr-OBu^t
Temperature (°C)   12
Calcium   7 mM
Substrate   5.7% (w/v) SCI (ge)
Enzyme   0.28, 0.43% (w/v) porcine trypsin TC

Analysis
Sampling (h)   24, 48, 72, 96, 168
Preparation   Acetone precipitation
Method   HPLC, gradient elution

Table 69 Yields of HI-OMe (α), DAI (α_1) and DOI plus DOI-Thr-OMe (β) in transpeptidation reactions using different proteases

	Bovine trypsin			Succinylated trypsin			A. lyticus protease		
H_2O (%)	19.7			19.7			26.0		
Temp. (°C)	4			4			4		
Time (h)	α	α_1	β*	α	α_1	β*	α	α_1	β
4	0	0	0	0	0	0	0	0	0
24	3	0	0	7	1	0	0	0	0
96	11	0	0	24	2	3	2	0	0
Temp. (°C)	12			12			12		
Time (h)	α	α_1	β*	α	α_1	β*	α	α_1	β
4	0	0	0	4	0	0	0	0	0
24	10	0	0	25	2	5	6	1	0
96	27	2	25	47	4	22	32	5	0
Temp. (°C)	25			25			25		
Time (h)	α	α_1	β*	α	α_1	β*	α	α_1	β
4	5	0	0	4	11	0	3	2	0
24	21	1	0	39	3	6	31	4	0
48	—	—	—	—	—	—	52	6	0
96	35	2	20	48	2	18	74	10	0
120	—	—	—	—	—	—	77	8	0

* Separation of SCI and DOI-Thr-OMe not achieved when large amounts of unconverted SCI are present

Conditions

Organic solvent	DMSO/BD 1/1 (v/v)
H_2O, % nominal	19.7, 26.0
Buffer (M/M)	HOAc/OAc⁻ 1.5/1
Threonine ester	1 M Thr-OMe
Temperature (°C)	4, 12, 25
Calcium	4 mM
Substrate	0.5% (w/v) SCI (ss)
Enzyme	0.25% (w/v) A. lyticus protease
	0.75% (w/v) bovine trypsin TC
	0.65% (w/v) succinylated porcine trypsin

Analysis

Sampling (h)	4, 24, 48, 96, 120
Preparation	Acetone precipitation
Method	HPLC, isocratic elution

Table 70 Yields of HI-OMe (α), DAI (α₁) and DOI plus DOI-Thr-OMe (β) in transpeptidation reactions

	A. lyticus protease						Succinylated trypsin					
H_2O (%)	21.4			28.6			21.4			28.6		
$HOAc/OAc^-$ (M/M)	0/1.11			1.67/1.11			0/1.11			1.67/1.11		
Time (h)	α	α₁	β	α	α₁	β	α	α₁	β	α	α₁	β*
24	28	0	0	2	0	0	0	0	0	25	3	0
48	46	0	0	10	0	0	0	0	0	32	3	0
72	56	2	0	17	0	0	0	0	0	33	3	0

* DOI-Thr-OMe is not detectable in the presence of large amounts of unconverted SCI

Conditions

Organic solvent	DMAC
H_2O, % nominal	21.4, 28.6
Buffer (M/M)	$HOAc/OAc^-$ 1.67/1.11, 0/1.11
Threonine ester	1.11 M Thr-OMe
Temperature (°C)	25
Calcium	8 mM
Substrate	0.6% (w/v) SCI (ss)
Enzyme	0.6% (w/v) succinylated porcine trypsin
	0.25% (w/v) A. lyticus protease

Analysis

Sampling (h)	24, 48, 72
Preparation	Acetone precipitation
Method	HPLC, isocratic elution

Table 71 Yields of HI-OBuᵗ (α) in transpeptidation reactions

	Porcine trypsin						Succinylated trypsin		
Trypsin (%) (w/v)	1.0			0.5			0.5		
Temp. (°C)	12	20	28	12	20	28	12	20	28
Time (h)	α	α	α	α	α	α	α	α	α
24	22	24	25	13	24	14	2	2	0
48	35	23	27	20	30	15	3	2	0

Conditions

Organic solvent	DMAC
H_2O, % nominal	19.8
Buffer (M/M)	$HOAc/OAc^-$ 0.125/1
Threonine ester	1 M Thr-OBuᵗ
Temperature (°C)	12, 20, 28
Calcium	4 mM
Substrate	0.5% (w/v) SCI (ss)
Enzyme	1%, 0.5% (w/v) porcine trypsin TC
	0.5% (w/v) succinylated porcine trypsin

Analysis

Sampling (h)	24, 48
Preparation	Acetone precipitation
Method	HPLC, gradient elution

Table 72 Yields of HI-OR (α), DAI (α_1), DOI (β_1), DOI-Thr-OR (β_2) and intermediate products (γ) in transpeptidation reactions of 3 single-chain insulin precursors

SCI

Thr-OR	Thr-OMe										Thr-OBu^t							
HOAc/OAc$^-$ (M/M); % H$_2$O, K.F.	1.70/1.14; 20.75					0/1.14; 19.66					1.70/1.14; 21.54				0/1.14; 22.38			
Time (h)	α	α_1	β_1	β_2	γ	α	α_1	β_1	β_2	γ	α	$\alpha_1\beta_2$*	β_1	γ	α	$\alpha_1\beta_2$*	β_1	γ
3.5	5	0	5**	†	—	15	0	3**	†	—	14	1	2	—	50	4	1	—
24	33	1	3	†	—	58	1	2	†	—	61	11	1	—	75	21	4	—
96	61	2	1	†	—	74	1	0	15	—	69	26	3	—	42	52	6	—
k(h^{-1})	0.015					0.046					0.043				0.20			

SCI-AAK***

Thr-OR	Thr-OMe										Thr-OBu^t							
HOAc/OAc$^-$ (M/M); % H$_2$O, K.F.	1.70/1.14; 20.28					0/1.14; 20.40					1.70/1.14; 22.31				0/1.14; 22.11			
Time (h)	α	α_1	β_1	β_2	γ	α	α_1	β_1	β_2	γ	α	$\alpha_1\beta_2$*	β_1	γ‡	α	$\alpha_1\beta_2$*	β_1	γ‡
3.5	17	0	0	†	0	51	0	0	†	0	25	3	0	2	42	2	0	5
24	60	2	1	†	0	86	2	2	5	0	61	6	1	1	72	4	1	2
96	84	2	1	4	0	87	2	2	9	0	82	9	2	0	89	8	3	0
k(h^{-1})††	0.053					0.20					0.082				0.16			

SCI-SK

Thr-OR	Thr-OMe										Thr-OBu^t							
HOAc/OAc$^-$ (M/M); % H$_2$O, K.F.	1.70/1.14; 21.47					0/1.14; 21.08					1.70/1.14; 22.55				0/1.14; 22.45			
Time (h)	α	α_1	β_1	β_2	γ	α	α_1	β_1	β_2	γ	α	$\alpha_1\beta_2$*	β_1	γ	α	$\alpha_1\beta_2$*	β_1	γ
3.5	27	0	0	1	26‡‡	63	0	0	2	20‡‡	73	7	4	0	83	5	0	0
24	81	2	2	2	13‡‡	81	2	6	11	0	84	15	1	0	78	16	6	0
96	81	3	3	4	0	70	3	4	23	0	66	30	3	0	51	43	6	0
k(h^{-1})††	0.090					0.28					>0.37				>0.51			

*   DAI and DOI-Thr-OBu^t not separated
†   SCI, SCI-AAK, and DOI-Thr-OMe not separated
‡   Peak eluting between DAI and HI-OBu^t
** Impurity present in starting material eluting in position of DOI
†† k calculated for overall process, disregarding the intermediates
‡‡ Intermediate eluting just after HI-OMe
*** Peaks eluting just after SCI-AAK are possibly opened but not coupled intermediates. These were disregarded in the calculations

Conditions
Organic solvent   DMF
H$_2$O, % nominal 21.0
Buffer (M/M)   HOAc/OAc$^-$ 0/1.14, 1.70/1.14
Threonine ester   1.14 M Thr-OMe, 1.14 M Thr-OBu^t
Temperature (°C) 12
Calcium   7 mM
Substrate   5.7% (w/v) SCI (ge), 5.7% (w/v) SCI-AAK (ge), 5.7% (w/v) SCI-SK (ge)
Enzyme   0.57% (w/v) porcine trypsin TC

Analysis
Sampling (h)   3.5, 24, 96
Preparation   Acetone precipitation
Method   HPLC, gradient elution

Table 73   Yields of HI-OR (α), DAI (α_1), DOI (β_1), DOI-Thr-OR (β_2), and intermediates (γ)

Trypsin, % w/v	Thr-OMe														
	0.57					0.34					0.17				
Time (h)	α	α_1	β_1	β_2	γ	α	α_1	β_1	β_2	γ	α	α_1	β_1	β_2	γ
24	88	2	†	3	0	68	2	†	5	0	53	3	†	5	0
48	89	1	3	6	0	78	2	†	4	0	74	0	†	5	0
72	87	1	3	9	0	91	0	†	4	0	86	0	†	5	0

Trypsin, % w/v	Thr-OBu^t												
	0.57				0.34				0.17			
Time (h)	α	$\alpha_1\beta_2$*	β_1	γ‡	α	$\alpha_1\beta_2$*	β_2	γ‡	α	$\alpha_1\beta_2$*	β_1	γ‡
24	84	4	0	2	71	3	0	3	63	2	0	5
48	90	6	0	0	84	5	0	1	80	4	0	2
72	89	7	4	0	80	4	0	2	88	5	7	0

* DOI-Thr-OBu^t and DAI not separated
† DOI and SCI-AAK not separated
‡ Peak in position between DAI and HI-OBu^t

Conditions
Organic solvent	DMF
H_2O, % nominal	21.0
Buffer (M/M)	HOAc/OAc$^-$ 0/1.14
Threonine ester	1.14 M Thr-OMe
Temperature (°C)	12
Calcium	7 mM
Substrate	5.7% (w/v) SCI-AAK (ge)
Enzyme	0.57, 0.34, 0.17% (w/v) porcine trypsin TC

Analysis
Sampling (h)	24, 48, 72
Preparation	Acetone precipitation
Method	HPLC, gradient elution

Table 74 Yields of HI-OMe (α), DAI (α_1), DOI (β_1), DOI-Thr-OMe (β_2), and intermediates in transpeptidation of SCI-AAK (γ). Difference to 100% accounted for by unconverted SCI-AAK

	1.14 M Thr-OMe									
H_2O (%)	20.0					21.0				
Time (h)	α	α_1	β_1	β_2	γ	α	α_1	β_1	β_2	γ
2	25	0	0	*	11	27	0	0	*	11
4	38	0	0	*	6	42	0	0	*	6
24	70	2	2	*	2	76	2	2	*	1
48	78	5	6	5	1	79	5	5	5	0
120	81	3	3	7	1	82	3	3	7	0
$k(\text{h}^{-1})$	0.14					0.16				
	0.57 M Thr-OMe									
H_2O (%)	20.0					21.0				
Time (h)	α	α_1	β_1	β_2	γ	α	α_1	β_1	β_2	γ
2	34	0	0	*	9	34	0	0	*	8
4	47	1	0	1	8	47	1	0	*	8
24	76	3	3	*	1	78	3	2	*	2
48	75	6	6	*	0	79	5	6	*	0
120	78	3	8	5	0	78	4	7	6	0
$k(\text{h}^{-1})$	0.22					0.22				

* DOI-Thr-OMe not separated from SCI-AAK

Conditions
Organic solvent DMF
H_2O, % nominal 20, 21
Buffer (M/M) HOAc/OAc$^-$ 0/0.57, 0/1.14
Threonine ester 0.57 M Thr-OMe, 1.14 M Thr-OMe
Temperature (°C) 8
Calcium 7 mM
Substrate 5.7% (w/v) SCI-AAK (ge)
Enzyme 0.57% (w/v) porcine trypsin TC

Analysis
Sampling (h) 2, 4, 24, 48, 72, 120
Preparation Acetone precipitation
Method HPLC, gradient elution

Table 75 Yields of HI-OMe (α), DAI (α_1), DOI (β_1), and DOI-Thr-OMe (β_2) in transpeptidation reactions using SCI-AAK as substrate. All unknown peaks between SCI-AAK and HI-OMe were included in the calculation of intermediates (γ)

H_2O (%), nominal H_2O (%) K.F. analysis		20.9 20.99					21.4 21.44					21.9 21.97			
Time (h)	α	α_1	β_1	β_2	γ	α	α_1	β_1	β_2	γ	α	α_1	β_1	β_2	γ
23	60	0	0	*	4	60	0	0	*	4	73	2	0	*	4
48	78	2	1	*	3	79	2	1	*	2	84	3	1	*	1
68	84	4	1	*	2	85	3	1	*	1	87	3	2	3	1

H_2O (%) nominal H_2O (%) K.F. analysis		22.4 22.48					22.9 22.69					23.4 22.90			
Time (h)	α	α_1	β_1	β_2	γ	α	α_1	β_1	β_2	γ	α	α_1	β_1	β_2	γ
23	77	2	1	*	3	78	1	1	*	2	77	1	1	*	2
48	86	3	2	3	1	87	4	2	3	1	86	3	2	4	1
68	89	3	2	3	0.5	89	3	2	4	0.5	90	3	2	4	0.5

* DOI-Thr-OMe coelutes with SCI-AAK

Conditions
Organic solvent   DMAC
H_2O, % nominal   20.9, 21.4, 21.9, 22.4, 22.9, 23.4
Buffer (M/M)   HOAc/OAc$^-$ 0/1.14
Threonine ester   1.14 M Thr-OMe
Temperature (°C)   12
Calcium   7 mM
Substrate   5.7% (w/v) SCI-AAK (ge)
Enzyme   0.57% (w/v) porcine trypsin TC

Analysis
Sampling (h)   23, 48, 68
Preparation   Acetone precipitation
Method   HPLC, isocratic elution

Table 76 First-order rate constants normalized to 1 mM trypsin for eight different reactions

Experiment	Reaction	Trypsin concentrations (mM)					Mean ± SD	Gross mean ± SD
		0.2	0.1	0.05	0.025	0.0125		k/T (min^{-1} mM^{-1})
		k/T (min^{-1} mM^{-1})						
8/2 -83	IA → IM	0.0165	0.0128	0.0133		0.0125	0.0138 ± 0.0018	
15/3 -83	IA → IM	0.0124					0.0124 ± 0.0009*	
15/3 -83	IA → IM	0.0157					0.0157 ± 0.0002*	
13/12-80	IA → IM	0.0177						
6/8 -85	IA → IM	0.0149					0.0149 ± 0.0011*	
27/4 -82	IA → IM	0.0142						
11/6 -82	IA → IM	0.0148						0.0142 ± 0.0019
20/2 -86	IA → IB	0.041					0.041 ± 0.004*	0.041 ± 0.004
31/10-85	IThr → IM	0.0118					0.0118 ± 0.0000†	0.0118
3/9 -85	IA → IM + IB	0.0299					0.0299 ± 0.0019†	0.0299 ± 0.0019
10/2 -83	I → IM		1.14	1.24	1.20	1.32		
7/1 -81	I → IM	1.38					1.23 ± 0.08	
3/9 -81	I → IM			1.46	1.37			
27/4 -82	I → IM	0.78						
11/6 -82	I → IM	0.83						1.19 ± 0.24
31/7 -85	IM → IB	0.240					0.240 ± 0.022*	0.240 ± 0.022
7/1 -81	I → IB	0.77						
17/3 -83	I → IB		0.52	0.43	0.52	0.40	0.47 ± 0.06	
28/10-81	I → IB	0.53	0.30	0.43	0.63		0.47 ± 0.15	
30/7 -85	I → IB	0.72					0.72 ± 0.04‡	0.50 ± 0.14
5/4 -83	I → IM + IB		1.38	1.33	1.43	1.50	1.41 ± 0.07	1.41 ± 0.07

* Results from experiments where concentrations of insulin compounds were varied. Average of four determinations using 2, 4, 6, and 8 mM insulin compound

† Average of three determinations, see Tables 33 and 38

‡ Experiment in 22% H$_2$O, cf. Table 37. Data excluded from gross mean

Conditions: 20.7% water in DMAC, 1 M Thr-OR, HOAC/OAc$^-$ = 1.5/1 (M/M) and 12°C. Rate constants determined as $-\ln(S/100)/t$ where S is percentage unconverted insulin substrate determined by HPLC

Table 77 First-order rate constants for release of alanine from porcine insulin in various amines normalized to 1 mM trypsin

Experiment	Reaction	Amine	k/T (min^{-1} mM^{-1})	Mean ± SD
13/5-81	IA → IM	Thr-OMe	0.013	
21/5-81	IA → IM		0.011	
9/6-81	IA → IM		0.016*	
24/7-81	IA → IM		0.015*	
29/7-81	IA → IM		0.013	0.0136 ± 0.0019
21/5-81	IA → IB	Thr(Bu^t)-OBu^t	0.049	
21/5-81	IA → IM + IB	Thr-OMe + Thr(Bu^t)-OBu^t	0.024	
3/6-81	IA → I	N(Et)$_3$	0.006	
9/6-81	IA → I		0.011†	0.09
13/5-81	IA → I	NMM	0.039	
29/7-81	IA → I	N(CH$_3$)$_4$-OH	0.021	

* HPLC analysis of IM formation superimposable
† Fresh bottle of N(Et)$_3$

Conditions: 20.7% water in DMAC, 1 M amine, HOAc/OAc$^-$ = 1.5/1 (M/M), temp. = 12°C, using 0.2 mM trypsin. Rate constants determined as $-\ln((100 - \%\text{Ala released})/100)/t$ where % Ala released represents the percentage alanine released from porcine insulin